W0050535

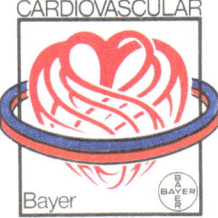

Th. v. Arnim / A. Maseri (Eds.)

Predisposing Conditions for Acute Ischemic Syndromes

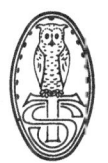 Springer-Verlag Berlin Heidelberg GmbH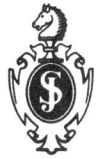

Priv.-Doz. Dr. med. Th. v. Arnim
Chefarzt der I. Med. Klinik
der Krankenanstalten Rotes Kreuz
Nymphenburger Str. 163
8000 München 19

Dr. A. Maseri
Cardiovascular Unit
Royal Postgraduate Medical School
Hammersmith Hospital
Ducane Road
London W12 OHS

The publication of this volume has been made possible by a grant from Bayer AG, Leverkusen

CIP-Titelaufnahme der Deutschen Bibliothek

Predisposing conditions for acute ischemic syndromes /
Th. v. Arnim; A. Maseri (eds.). — Darmstadt: Steinkopff; New York: Springer, 1989
   ISBN 978-3-662-09436-5   ISBN 978-3-662-09434-1 (eBook)
   DOI 10.1007/ 978-3-662-09434-1
NE: Arnim, Thomas von [Hrsg.]

Preface

"Predisposing conditions for acute ischemic syndromes" contains the proceedings of a conference held in Garmisch-Partenkirchen, West Germany, October 14 and 15, 1988.

The editors of this volume are most grateful to the authors for their effort to provide manuscripts before the meeting, to the sponsor, Bayer AG, for their generous support, and to the publishers for the efficient collaboration, all of which have made the appearance of this book possible. All authors contributed their manuscripts in advance and they are combined with an edited version of the discussions to allow rapid publication.

In coronary heart disease the prognosis for patients is largely determined by the occurrence of irreversible ischemic damage to the myocardium. Irreversible events are certainly preceded by a destabilization of a former stable situation. This destabilization may occur with increasing symptomatology or without apparent warning signs to patient and physician; it may occur over a longer time period or very suddenly. The statement, however, holds true that no patient has ever died from stable angina pectoris. Thus, if the prognosis for patients with ischemic heart disease is to be improved, the focus has to be set on recognition and treatment of unstable ischemic syndromes. It was the goal of the conference to gather scientists and clinicans from different fields of research, to get an up-to-date view of the different aspects of unstable ischemic syndromes and to foster interdisciplinary discussions.

Circadian variations have been shown to occur for transient ischemic episodes as well as for the occurrence of acute myocardial infarction and sudden death. Therefore, insight into the physiology of circadian rhythms may contain important clues about trigger mechanisms. Circumstantial evidence correlates psychosocial precursors with unstable ischemic syndromes, however, cause and effect relations remain a matter of discussion. Changes in the fibrinolytic system, platelet reactivity, or blood hemorheology may all contribute to destabilization of a stable pattern of ischemia.

The most striking evidence connects acute alterations in an atherosclerotic plaque, such as fissure, thrombus formation and subintimal hematoma, to acute changes in symptomatology and severity of ischemic heart disease. The pathologic and angiographic changes therefore deserve concentrated attendance and must be correlated with clinical information, be it symptomatic alteration of the patient or objective signs of ischemia or other markers without symptoms.

If predisposing conditions for acute ischemic syndromes can be identified, the preventive treatment to avoid irreversible damage is the desired consequence. Obviously, strategies to lower risk factors are most important, but in later stages of the disease interventional techniques come into play. Drug treatment has shown preventive efficacy for, for instance, aspirin and others, such as calcium antagonists, are under intensive study.

Th. v. Arnim, Munich
A. Maseri, London

Contents

Circadian variations in the effects of cardiovascular active drugs

B. Lemmer

Zentrum der Pharmakologie, J. W. Goethe-Universität, Frankfurt, FRG

Introduction

It is now well established that all functions of the cardiovascular system display significant circadian variations (for review see [13 - 15]). Actually, biological rhythms in heart rate and blood pressure were described at the end of the 18th and the beginning of the 19th centuries. Falconer in 1797 described periodicities in pulse rate and mentioned that "the pulse, even in the state of perfect health, varies considerably at different times of day" [8]. Similarly, in 1801, Autenrieth described in his "Handbuch der empirischen menschlichen Physiologie" that the pulse was slower in the morning than in the evening and that daily changes occurred also in body temperature [4]. A daily variability in blood pressure was reported by Zadek in 1881 [35] and by Hill in 1898 [10]. Following these early reports, numerous more sophisticated studies have provided additional convincing evidence for circadian rhythms in heart rate and in systolic and diastolic blood pressure, both in healthy subjects and in patients suffering from cardiovascular diseases (for review see [13—17]).

Though the rhythms in heart rate and blood pressure are the most well known periodic functions within the cardiovascular system other parameters have been shown to exhibit circadian variations as well (Fig. 1), e.g., in blood flow, stroke volume, capillary resistance, parameters of ECG recordings, in the plasma concentrations of noradrenaline, cAMP (Fig. 2), renin, angiotensin, aldosterone and atrial natriuretic hormone, in blood viscosity and aggregability, etc. (see [13—15]). These findings clearly demonstrate a pronounced rhythmic circadian organization of the cardiovascular system as well as of the mechanisms involved in its regulation.

Aside from circadian rhythms in physiological functions of the cardiovascular system, various clinical reports also indicate the onset of cardiovascular diseases, and symptoms exhibit a pronounced temporal dependency (for review see [13—17]). Some representative data are summarized in Fig. 3. It is interesting to note that in patients suffering from angina pectoris ST-segment elevations occur more frequently at night ([1], see also Fig. 3), whereas ST-Segment depressions are registered more often during daytime hours [2], indicating differences in etiology.

Taking all these data together it is not surprising to note that the effects, as well as the pharmacokinetics of drugs used in the treatment of cardiovascular disorders, were shown to display circadian variations. This will be demonstrated in some representative examples.

1

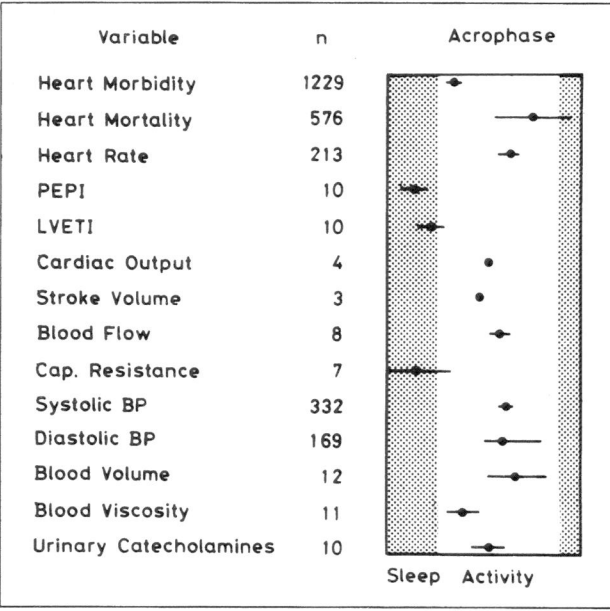

Variable	n	Acrophase
Heart Morbidity	1229	
Heart Mortality	576	
Heart Rate	213	
PEPI	10	
LVETI	10	
Cardiac Output	4	
Stroke Volume	3	
Blood Flow	8	
Cap. Resistance	7	
Systolic BP	332	
Diastolic BP	169	
Blood Volume	12	
Blood Viscosity	11	
Urinary Catecholamines	10	

Sleep   Activity

Fig. 1 Acrophase (time of peak value of rhythm) map in cardiovascular functions in man. (Adapted from [32]: from [15])

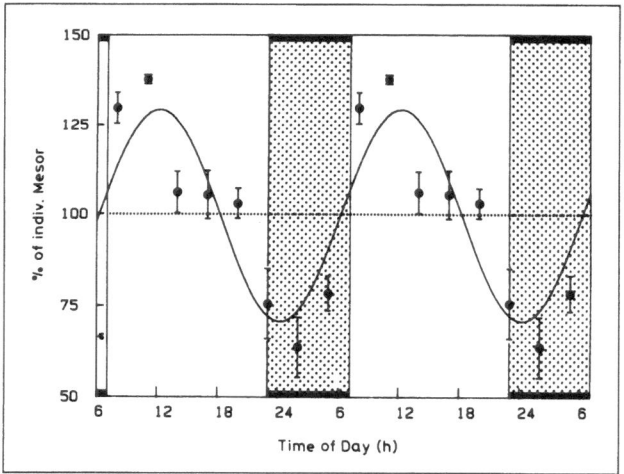

Fig. 2. Circadian rhythm in plasma cAMP content of healthy subjects. Percent of variation around the 24-h-mean, mean ± SEM, n=6; double plot. (From Lemmer and Witte, unpublished results)

Chronopharmacology of cardiovascular active drugs

Beta-adrenoceptor blocking drugs: beta-receptor blocking drugs are of great therapeutic value in the treatment of various cardiovascular disorders, e.g., coronary heart disease, hypertension, and arrhythmias. This group of drugs has been intensively studied in animal experiments [16, 19, 22] as well as in patients in relation

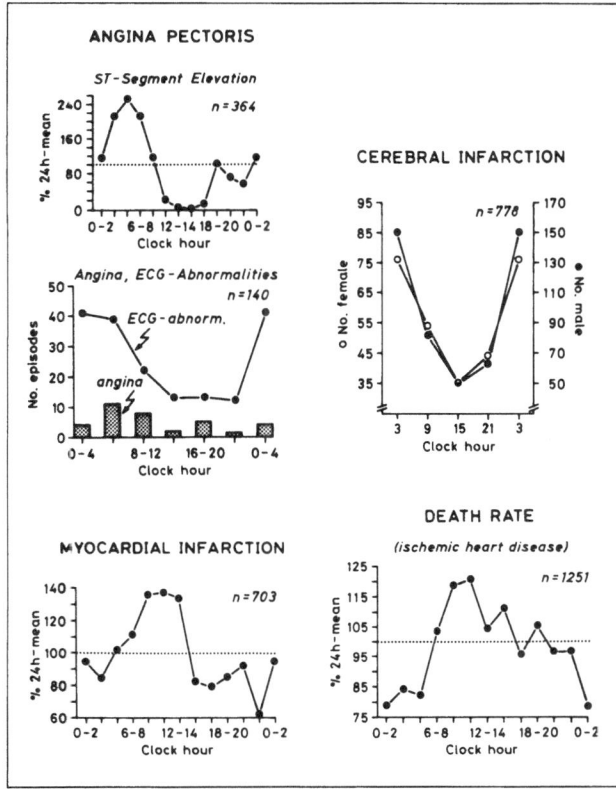

Fig. 3. Summary of circadian-stage-dependent pathophysiological findings in cardiovascular diseases. *Angina pectoris*: ST-segment elevation in 25 patients with variant angina pectoris (upper part; [1]); angina attacks and ECG-abnormalities such as ST-segment elevation, ST-segment depression, or T-wave pseudonormalization in 13 patients with variant angina pectoris (lower part; [33]). *Myocardial infarction*: onset evaluated by the MB-creatinase method in 703 patients [26]. *Cerebral infarction*: evaluated in 778 male and female patients [23]. *Death rate*: evaluated in 1 251 patients for ischemic heart disease [25]. (Adapted from [17])

[29, 14, 15] to circadian time. The various beta-receptor blocking drugs differ not only in their specific effects (receptor affinity and selectivity, intrinsic sympathomimetic activity), but also in their non-specific effects, which are related to the lipophilicity of the respective compound. Furthermore, the beta-receptor blocking drugs differ greatly in their main routes of elimination; lipophilic compounds are mainly biotransformed in the liver, whereas the hydrophilic ones are eliminated mainly in unchanged form by the kidneys. Since the functions of both these organs exhibit 24 h bioperiodicities [13, 15], differences in the drugs' pharmacokinetics have to be considered. However, chronopharmacokinetic studies with beta-blockers differing in the above mentioned properties have only been performed in rats [9, 22]. In man only the pharmacokinetics of propranolol were investigated at different times of day [12]. Significant daily variations in pharmacokinetic parameters were found with peak values in Cmax, absorption rate, AUC, and shortest elimination half-life after drug intake at 0800 hrs ([12] see Fig. 4). Interestingly, the stereospecific metabolism of propranolol did not display a circadian-phase-dependency [12].

Considerably more data are available on the circadian-stage-dependency of the cardiovascular effects of beta-receptor blocking drugs. Various groups have convincingly demonstrated that beta-receptor blocking drugs when taken regularly re-

3

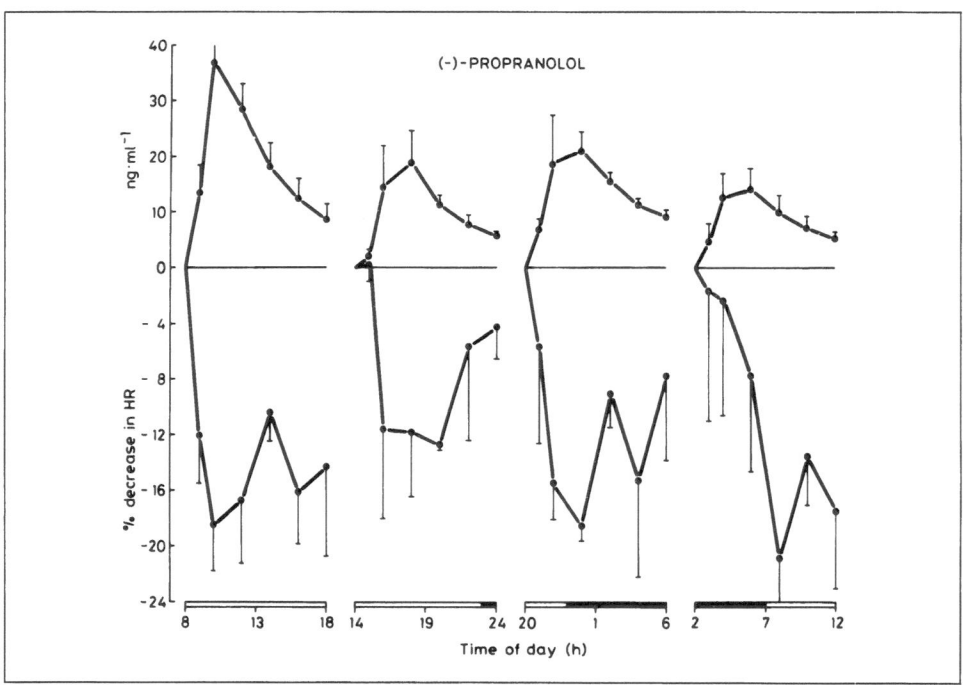

Fig. 4. Circadian-phase-dependency of the plasma concentrations of (—)-propranolol and the heart rate lowering as percentage of circadian control values. Mean ± SEM of four healthy volunteers who took 80 mg racemic propranolol p.o. either at 0800, 1400, 2000 or at 0200 hrs, resp. (From [12])

duce high blood pressure and heart rate in hypertensive patients more profoundly during the day than during the night (for review see [15]; Fig. 5). This circadian pattern in drug effects was, in general, observed with all the different beta-blockers, independently whether lipophilic (e.g., propranolol, oxprenolol) or hydrophilic (e.g., atenolol), whether non-selective (e.g., propranolol, oxprenolol, pindolol) or relative β_1-selective (e.g., atenolol, metoprolol) compounds were applied, or whether the drugs are known to be eliminated mainly by hepatic metabolism (lipophilic ones) or by renal excretion (hydrophilic ones) (for review see [14, 15]. Similar circadian-stage-dependent effects of propranolol were described after a single oral application of propranolol to healthy subjects [12]. Figure 4 demonstrates that the changes in heart rate in relation to the corresponding circadian control values were markedly different depending on the time of propranolol ingestion. The most interesting finding of this study was that after administration of propranolol at 0200 hrs the heart rate was only slightly affected within the first six hours after drug intake. However, two hours later, at the onset of the activity span when sympathetic tone was increasing again (see Fig. 2), the heart-rate-lowering effect was marked again and about equal to that found after drug application at 0800 hrs (Fig. 4). Plasma concentrations of propranolol at these two time points, on the other hand, differed by about a factor of 3 (Fig. 4).

4

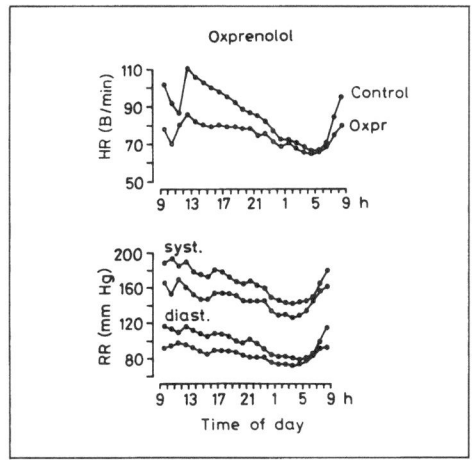

Fig. 5 Circadian rhythms in heart rate (HR) and blood pressure (RR) in 20 hypertensive patients before and after six weeks of chronic treatment with the beta-blocker oxprenolol. (Adapted from [29])

From the cardiovascular findings on beta-receptor blockade described it is already obvious that the chronokinetics of the drugs may not explain the more pronounced cardiovascular effects which occur during the activity period of both man and rat. It was, therefore, assumed that these rhythms may be due to rhythmic changes in vascular reactivity and sympathetic tone [12, 22]. In support of this hypothesis biochemical studies in rat heart ventricles and in rat forebrain revealed pronounced temporal variation in the basal level of the second messenger cAMP as well as in the activities of the enzymes involved in its formation (adenylate cyclase) and hydrolysis (phosphodiesterase), whereas beta-receptor affinity or number did not vary at all or only slightly varied with time of day [18, 21]. Results of a representative study are shown in Fig. 6.

Circadian-stage-dependent effects of propranolol have also been described in patients with stable angina pectoris [11]. Under control conditions as well as under treatment with propranolol, maximum increase in heart rate and ST-segment depression occurred when exercise was performed at 1600 hrs rather than at 0800 and 1200 hrs (Fig. 7), indicating that exercise is better tolerated in the afternoon than in the early morning. These results suggest that myocardial oxygen supply and oxygen demand are also subject to circadian variation.

Calcium channel blockers: calcium channel blockers (calcium antagonists) are used in the treatment of coronary heart disease and of hypertension. Drugs such as verapamil, diltiazem, nifedipine and nitrendipine decrease the free intracellular calcium concentration in the heart leading to a reduction in oxygen demand. They also have a relaxing effect on smooth muscle. Calcium channel blockers of the verapamil-type and diltiazem have a more prominent cardiac, i.e., negativ chronotropic effect, whereas those of the dihydropyridine-type (nifedipine, nitrendipine) have a more dominant vasodilating effect. With the latter compounds even a reflexly induced increase in heart rate can be observed. Chronopharmacological studies in hypertensive patients have shown that, in general, the blood pressure lowering effect of these

5

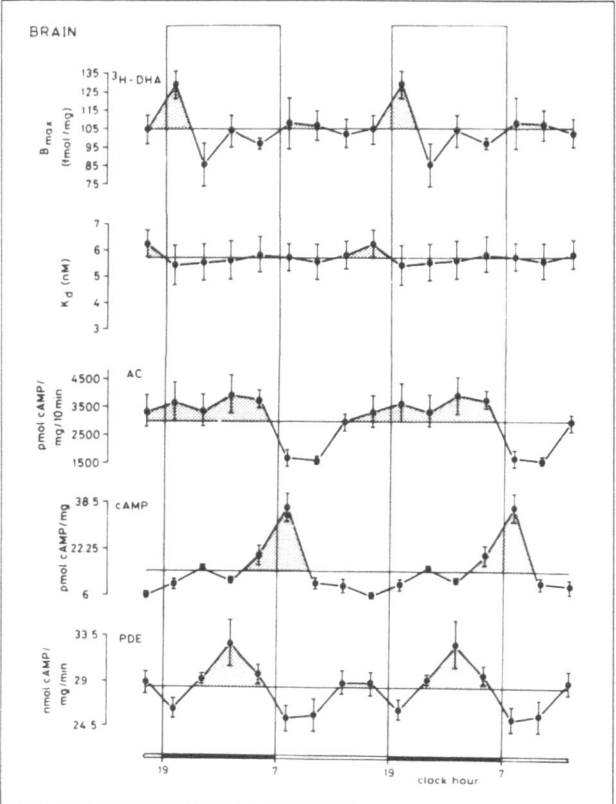

Fig. 6. Daily variations in the beta-adrenoceptor — adenylate cyclase (AC) — cAMP — phosphodiesterase (PDE) — system in rat forebrain. Bmax- and Kd-values were determined in saturation experiments with ^{3}H-DHA. Dark phase from 1900—7000 hrs, means ± SEM, n = 4—8, double plot. (Data from [18])

drugs was more marked during daytime than during night [9, 15, 17]. More interestingly, the differences in the predominant site of action of the two groups of calcium channel blockers (cardiac vs vascular) can clearly be observed in their effects on the circadian rhythm in heart rate: whereas verapamil reduced heart rate significantly during daytime hours, nifedipine had no effect on heart rate, and nitrendipine even increased heart rate during early morning hours [17].

Other drugs: chronic treatment of hypertensive patients with clonidine applied by a transdermal disk reduced blood pressure during the daytime [30]; no measurements were reported at night.

After a combined treatment with methyldopa and a diuretic the circadian rhythm in blood pressure was preserved, although the 24-h-level was reduced relative to the pretreatment value [6].

Alpha-adrenoceptor blocking drugs such as indoramine and prazosin had quite similar effects on the circadian rhythms in blood pressure and heart rate as already described for beta-blockers [17].

Diuretics are among the drugs of first choice in the treatment of hypertension. They are known to decrease peripheral vascular resistance by inhibiting sodium retention. The antihypertensive effects of xipamide has been studied after chronic dosing in hypertensive patients [28]. Xipamide reduced the level of elevated blood pressure throughout 24 h. The fact that this diuretic also reduced the early morning rise in blood pressure may explain why a consistent 24-h decrease in high blood pressure has been described for combined treatment with beta-blocking drugs and diuretics [15].

Recently, converting enzyme inhibitors such as captopril in combination with a diuretic were also shown to affect high blood pressure more pronouncedly during daytime hours than during night [3, 24, 27].

Antianginal drugs: As already mentioned in patients suffering from variant angina pectoris the onset and the frequency of angina attacks exhibit a circadian rhythm (Fig. 3). On the other hand, angina attacks in connection with ST-segment depression are more frequent during daytime [2]. It is, therefore, not surprising that antianginal drugs may also exert circadian-phase-dependent effects. First evidence for this was provided by the classical report of Yasue et al. [34]: the authors demonstrated a nitroglycerine-induced increase in the patency of the great coronary arteries, when the drug was taken in the morning but not when taken in the afternoon (Fig. 8). Similar findings in patients with stable angina pectoris without and with treatment by propranolol were mentioned above (see Fig. 7).

The chronopharmacology of the oral nitrates isosorbide dinitrate (ISDN) and isosorbide-5-mononitrate (IS-5-MN) has been investigated only in preliminary studies in healthy subjects ([5, 20, 31], and unpublished results). Maximum in ISDN-

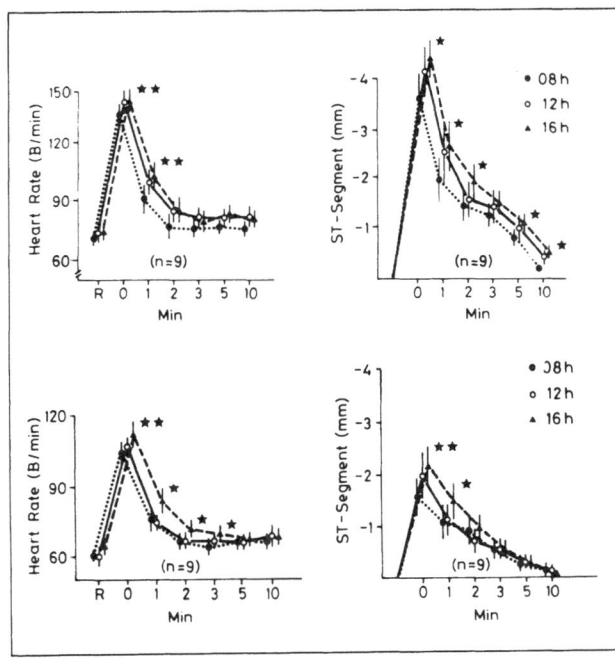

Fig. 7. Circadian-stage-dependency in exercise-limited increase in heart rate and ST-segment depression in nine Caucasian patients with stable angina pectoris without (upper part) or with chronic therapy with propranolol (lower part). Exercise was performed at 0800, 1200 or at 1600 hrs, respectively. * $p < 0.05$; ** $p < 0.025$ For 1600 to 0800 hrs exercise. (Adapted from [11])

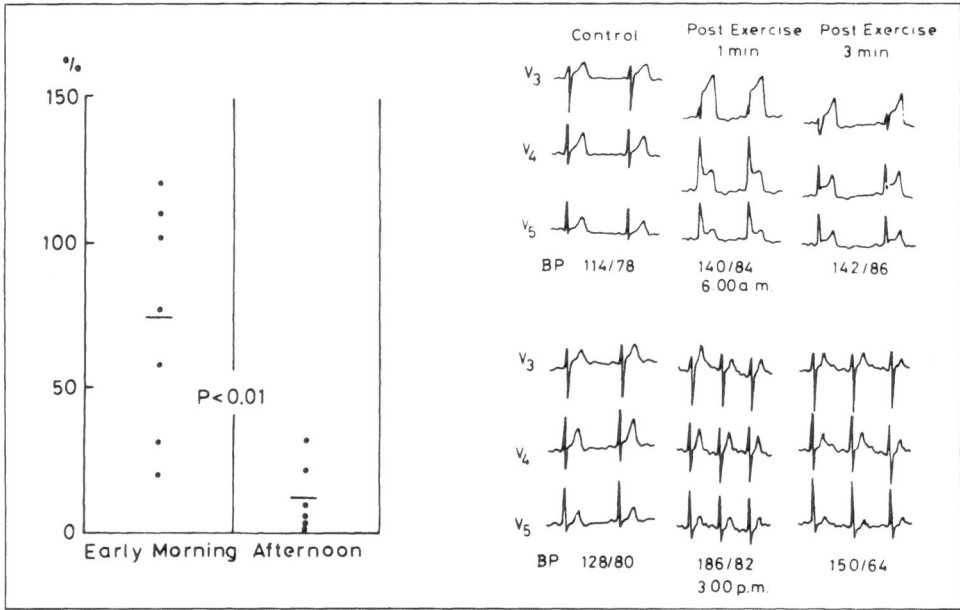

Fig. 8. Circadian-stage-dependency in exercise ECG (left part, one patient) and glyceroltrinitrate-induced increase in coronary artery diameter (right part, 13 patients) in patients with Prinzmetal angina pectoris. (Adapted from [34])

induced decrease in blood pressure and increase in heart rate were found after night-time dosing [20]. Daily variations were also seen in the pharmacokinetics of an immediate-release preparation of IS-5-MN with Tmax being 0.9 and 2.1 h at drug intake at 0630 hrs and 1830 hrs, respectively [31]. In contrast, decrease in blood pressure and increase in heart rate occurred ab about 0.6—1.0 h after drug ingestion at either dosing time, thus, giving evidence for a dissociation in time between peak drug concentrations and peak effects during the evening hours ([31], unpublished). Similar results were obtained after oral dosing of a IS-5-MN retard formulation either at 0800 hrs or at 2000 hrs. Maximum decrease in standing blood pressure and increase in heart rate occurred about 3 hours after drug intake at 2000 hrs, but about 5—6 h after drug intake at 0800 hrs. No circadian-phase-dependency was observed in the pharmacokinetics of this retard preparation. These data clearly demonstrate that the kind of drug formulation may also influence the pharmacokinetic profile of a drug when taken at different times of day.

Conclusion

The published data on the chronopharmacology of cardiovascular active drugs may have clinical implications. Firstly, these data demonstrate that the pharmacokinetics as well as the effects of these drugs are due to circadian variations. Furthermore, these findings, together with the rhythmic organization of all functions of the cardiovascular system, make the assumption unlikely that "therapeutic windows" in drug treatment really do exist. Recently published on heparin for findings obtained in patients with thromboembolism clearly demonstrate that treating in such a manner so as to achieve a constant drug level throughout 24 h may be unwise. In this study heparin was infused at a constant rate over 48 h [7]. Significant circadian rhythms in the anticoagulant effects of heparin were found with peak-to-trough variations in the range of 40—60% of the respective 24-h mean. Most important, the greatest anticoagulant effect reproducibly occurred early at night during each day of the 48-h infusion, at the time when bleeding was most often observed. Based on the chronopharmacological data available it is concluded that in addition to the physico-chemical properties of a drug, its dosage, pharmacokinetics, and galenic formulation, the additional parameter "time of day" has to be taken into account in order to increase the therapeutic range of a drug or in order to more appropriately treat the disease.

Acknowledgement: The author's studies were supported by grants from the Deutsche Forschungsgemeinschaft, Dr. Paul und Cilli-Weill Stiftung, Riese-Stiftung, und Scheidel-Stiftung.

References

1. Araki H, Koiwaya Y, Nakagaki O, Nakamura M (1983) Diurnal distribution of ST-segment elevation and related arrhythmias in patients with variant angina; a study by ambulatory ECG monitoring. Circulation 67: 995—1000
2. Arnim von T, Höfling B, Schreiber M (1985) Characteristics of episodes of ST elevation or ST depression during ambulatory monitoring in patients subsequently undergoing coronary angiography. Br Heart J 54: 484 — 488
3. Asmar RG, Pannier BM, Hugue ChJ, Laurent S, Safavian A, Safar ME (1987) Captopril + hydrochlorothiazide 24h ambulatory monitoring effects. Br J clin Pharmac 23: 77S—81 S
4. Autenrieth JHF (1801) Handbuch der empirischen Physiologie, Teil 1. Jakob Friedrich Heerbrandt, Tübingen
5. Blume H, Scheidel B, Becker HJ, Renczes J, Lemmer B (1986) Chronopharmacology of oral isosorbide dinitrate in healthy subjects. Naunyn-Schmiedeberg's Arch Pharmacol 332: R 57
6. Bock KD, Kreuzenbeck W (1966) Spontaneous blood pressure variations in hypertension; the effect of antihypertensive therapy and correlations with the incidence of complications. In: Gross F (ed) Antihypertensive Therapy. Springer-Verlag, Berlin, p 224—237
7. Decousus HA, Croze M, Levi FA, Jaubert JG, Perpoint BM, DeBonadonna JF, Reinberg, A, Queneau PM (1985) Circadian changes in anticoagulant effect of heparin infused at a constant rate. Br Med J 290: 341—344
8. Falconer W (1797) Beobachtungen über den Puls. JS Heinsius, Leipzig
9. Gould BA, Hornung RS, Mann S, Balasubramanian V, Raftery EB (1982) Slow channel inhibitors verapamil and nifedipine in the management of hypertension. J. Cardiovasc Pharmacol 4: 5369—5373
10. Hill L (1898) On rest, sleep and work and the concomittant changes in the circulation of the blood. Lancet 1: 282—288
11. Joy M, Pollard CM, Nunan TO (1982) Diurnal variation in exercise in angina pectoris. Br Heart J 48: 156—160
12. Langner B, Lemmer B (1988) Circadian changes in the pharmacokinetics and cardiovascular effects of oral propranolol in healthy subjects. Eur J. Clin Pharmacol 33: 619—624

13. Lemmer B (1984) Chronopharmakologie — Tagesrhythmen und Arzneimittelwirkung —. Wiss. Verlagsges., 2^{ne} ed 1984
14. Lemmer B (1986) The chronopharmacology of cardiovascular medications. Ann Rev Chronopharmacol 2: 199—258
15. Lemmer B (1987) Chronopharmacology of cardiovascular medications. In: Kuemmerle HP. Hitzenberger G, Spitzy KH (eds) Klinische Pharmakologie. ecomed Verlagsgesellschaft, Landsberg München, 4. Auflage, 12. Erg. Lfg. 11/87: 1—14
16. Lemmer B (1989) Temporal aspects in the effects of cardiovascular active drugs in man. In: Lemmer B (ed) Chronopharmacology: Cellular and Biochemical Interactions. Marcel Dekker Inc. New York Basel, in preparation
17. Lemmer B (1989) Cardiovascular system. In: Arendt J, Waterhouse J, Minors D (eds) Biological Rhythms in Clinical Practice. J Wright publ, Hertfordshire, in preparation
18. Lemmer B, Bärmeier H, Schmidt S, Lang P-H (1987b) On the daily variation in the beta-receptor — adenylate cyclase — cAMP — phosphodiesterase system in rat forebrain. Chronobiol Int 4: 469—475
19. Lemmer B, Bathe K, Lang P-H, Neumann G, Winkler H (1983) Chronopharmacology of β-adrenoceptor blocking drugs: Pharmacokinetics and pharmacodynamic studies in rats. J Am Coll Toxicol 2: 347—35
20. Lemmer B, Becker HJ, Renczes J, Scheidel B, Blume H (1986) Circadian-phase-dependency in the pharmacokinetics and cardiovascular effects of oral isosorbide dinitrate in man. Ann Rev Chronopharmacol 3: 339—342
21. Lemmer B, Lang P-H, Schmidt S, Bärmeier H (1987a) Evidence for circadian rhythmicity of the beta-adrenoceptor — adenylate cyclase — cAMP — phosphodiesterase system in the rat. J Cardiovasc Pharmacol 10: S138 — S140
22. Lemmer B, Winkler H, Ohm T and Fink M (1985) Chronopharmacokinetics of beta-receptor blocking drugs of different lipophilicity (propranolol, metoprolol, sotalol, atenolol) in plasma and tissues after single and multiple dosing in the rat. Naunyn-Schmiedeberg's Arch Pharmacol 330: 42 — 49
23. Marshall J (1977) Diurnal variation in occurrence of strokes. Stroke 8: 230—231
24. Meijer JL, Ardesch HG, Van Rooijen JC, De Bruijn JHB (1987) Captopril plus hydrochlorithiazide once daily normalizes 24h blood pressure in patients with essential hypertension. Br J clin Pharmac. 23: 83S—88S
25. Mitler MM, Hajdukovic RM, Shafor R, Hahn PM, Kripke DF (1987) When people die. Cause of death versus time of death. Am J Med 82: 266—274
26. Muller JE, Stone PH, Turin ZG, Rutherford JG, Czeisler CA, Parkers C, Poole WK, Passamani E, Roberts R, Robertson T, Sobel BE, Willerson JT; Braunwald E (1985) The Milis study group: Circadian variation in the frequency of onset of acute myocardial infarction. N Engl J Med 313: 1315—1322
27. Poggi L, Vaisse B, Bernard F, Drivet-Perrin J, Sambuc R (1987) Comparison of once and twice daily administration of captopril plus hydrochlorothiazide on 24h blood pressure levels. Br J clin Pharmac 23: 71S — 75S
28. Raftery EB, Melville DI, Gould BA, Mann S, Whittington JR (1981) A study of the antihypertensive action of xipamide using ambulatory intra-arterial monitoring. Br J Clin Pharmacol 12: 381—385
29. Raftery EB, Millar-Craig MW, Mann S, Balasubramanian V (1981) Effects of treatment on circadian rhythms of blood pressure. Biotelem Pat Monitor 8: 113—120
30. Schaller MD, Nussberger J, Waeber B, Porchet M, Brunner HR (1985) Transdermal clonidine therapy in hypertensive patients. JAMA 253: 233—235
31. Scheidel B, Blume H, Stenzhorn G, Lemmer B, Lenhard G (1987) Chronopharmacokinetics and chronohemodynamics of immediate-release isosorbide-5-mononitrate in man. Chronobiologia 14: 233
32. Smolensky MH, Tatar SE, Bergmann SA, Losman JG, Barnard CN, Dacso CC, Kraft IA (1976) Circadian rhythmic aspects of human cardiovascular function: a review by chronobiologic statistical methods. Chronobiologia 3: 337—371
33. Waters DD, Miller DD, Bouchard A, Bosch X, Theroux P (1984) Circadian variation in variant angina. Am J Cardiol 54: 61—64

34. Yasue H, Omote S, Takizawa A, Nagao M, Miwa K, Tanaka S (1979) Circadian variation of exercise capacity in patients with Prinzmetal's variant angina: role of exercise-induced coronary arterial spasm. Circulation 59: 938—948
35. Zadek J (1881) Die Messung des Blutdrucks des Menschen mittels des Bach'schen Apparates. Z Klin Med 2: 509—55

Author's address:
Prof. Dr. med. Björn Lemmer
Zentrum der Pharmakologie
J. W. Goethe-Universität
Theodor-Stern-Kai 7
D-6000 Frankfurt/M 70, FRG

Discussion

FOX:

In shift workers where you change the pattern, do the circadian variations that you mentioned alter automatically because you change the waking and sleeping hours?

LEMMER:

There has been some work done in shift workers, but as far as I know, no single work on drug effectiveness. We know that shift workers suffer, for example, from sleep disturbances and gastro-intestinal (GI) disturbances, and so on, but in no case were drug data taken on these shift workers. I think it is very important to look for these effects.

On the other hand, we know that in shift workers different circadian rhythms change with the type of the shift, so that we have the observation of an internal desynchronization in these people. Obviously this internal desynchronization contributes to the disenabling of different capabilities of the shift workers, quite similar to jet lag.

VON ARNIM:

You finished your talk by saying that we might better understand things. I think so far things are becoming more and more complicated. Let me ask a simple question regarding your data on pro-pranolol. Was it always one dose that the probands got at the different times of day?

LEMMER:

Yes, only a single dose at the different times of the day with a wash-out period of one week between each study.

VON ARNIM:

Effects went on much longer than the half-life of the drug level would have told us.

LEMMER:

This is not unusual, for we now know if measuring the binding, for example, on beta-receptors, that the half maximal effective dose is much lower than conventionally assumed. You could observe in our last study, which took place at 02.00 hr, that only one-third of the concentration led to the same effect as the three-fold dosage in the morning. So, the half maximal dosage of propranolol inhibiting the sympathetic tone is in the range of 10—15 mg.

GOHLKE:

Did you also do these very interesting studies in patients with coronary artery disease? There is evidence that some of the autonomic responses in patients with coronary artery disease might be blunted. There is an excellent study by Ellestad, who has shown that the heart-rate response to the Valsalva maneuver, to standing up, to similar actions, are markedly blunted in comparison to normals.

LEMMER:

Not until now. The reason is quite simple, for there were no published data either on the chrono-kinetic behavior of oral beta-blockers or of oral nitrates in human beings. So we at first started in healthy volunteers, but of course as we have the data in healthy human subjects, now we are going to see what the kinetics, as well as the effects, will be in patients at different times of day. I think it is very important to combine these studies, kinetics together with effects, and not only the one or the other. In all these studies there was a dissociation between the two functions, showing that the circadian rhythm in the regulation of the whole system is very important for the effect. This is under investigation.

MATHES:

From the absorption data, one would guess that the attenuation changes according to the activity of the sympathetic system. But from your dose that you give at 02.00 hr one also must see that absorption is not only less, but also slower than previously shown. Are there any further indications that this is true for other drugs as well, and that the GI-system also varies in terms of function during the day?

LEMMER:

Yes, there are quite a lot of data, but only with lipophilic compounds. Diazepam, propranolol, oral nitrates, and verapamil were shown to have either shorter T max when taken in the morning or higher C max as well as T max. So this indicates that absorption is more rapid in the morning than in the afternoon. Quite recently Moore from Utrecht could demonstrate that gastric emptying is more rapid in human beings in the morning than in late afternoon or at night. These data may represent differences in absorption time due to variations in gastric emptying. But this has only been shown for lipophilic compounds, not for hydrophilic cones. Even with theophyllin, there are similar findings of a longer time to peak concentration in the afternoon than when the drug is taken in the morning. This fits very nicely with the delay in gastric emptying.

MASERI:

There is a study by the World Health Organization published about seven or eight years ago which collected data about acute myocardial infarction in 14 cities in Europe and one city in Israel. They collected information over 7,000 patients and I think they were among the first to describe the circadian variation and the time of the day in which infarction was most prevalent. In some cities there was no definite trend, but in the majority, putting all the data together, there was a peak of about 35 % at about 10.00 hr. I think justice should be done to this study to be quoted about circadian occurrence of myocardial infarction.

FOX:

Was there a difference in the ethnic distribution that might have had a difference in the variation of the different cities?

MASERI:

No, the cities were all European except for one, which was in Israel.

LEMMER:

Well, at least in the seven or eight studies that I know, they all agree in that there is a prominent peak around 10.00 hr, and sometimes they found an additional peak at 20.00 hr. So, the dominant peak is in the morning, independent of location.

The treatment effects on circadian variation of transient myocardial ischemia

K. Fox, D. Mulcahy

National Heart Hospital, Westmoreland Street, London, England

Introduction

Considerable attention has been focused in recent times on the concept of silent myocardial ischemia, particularly as it is now clear that the majority of episodes of myocardial ischemia in patients with stable angina are asymptomatic [7]. Previous studies have shown a circadian pattern to these ischemic episodes with the peak occurring in the morning hours [6]. A similar circadian distribution has been reported for the occurrence of sudden death and acute myocardial infarction [2, 3]. This circadian distribution of acute myocardial infarction was apparently not seen in those patients receiving beta blocking drugs [2] but was unaltered in those receiving calcium antagonists [10].

The purpose of this report is to establish whether there is a circadian pattern of the total ischemic burden and to determine if this does correspond with the reported circadian pattern of acute myocardial infarction and sudden death. In particular, this study will investigate the effects of two drug treatments; the first a calcium channel blocker which will act by increasing myocardial oxygen supply as well as reducing myocardial oxygen demand, and a beta blocker which will act principally by reducing myocardial oxygen demand.

Patients and methods

One-hundred-fifty patients with angiographically documented coronary artery disease underwent ST segment monitoring off all routine anti-anginal medications; 6264 h of monitoring were performed in 121 men and 29 women (mean age 55 years); 46 Patients had single-vessel disease 37 two-vessel disease, and 67 three-vessel disease.

Fifty-three of these patients also underwent 48 h of ST segment monitoring while receiving either nifedipine (N = 12), atenolol (N = 20), or both nifedipine and atenolol at different times (N = 21). All 53 patients underwent ambulatory ST segment monitoring both off therapy and while on nifedipine (39—60 mg mean 45.5 mg daily) or atenolol (100 mg daily) as a part of various therapeutic trials. The drugs were administered double-blind and in a randomized fashion in all cases.

Ambulatory ST segment monitoring was performed using two bipolar leads (CM5 and inferior leads). Two-channel recordings were then obtained on a magnetic tape using a frequency modulated dual-channel recorder (Oxford Medilog II, frequency response 0.05—40 hertz). All tapes were visually analyzed at 60-times normal speed using an Oxford Medilog MA II scanner and all printouts were at 25 mm/s. ST segment depression was defined as planar or down-sloping ST segment shift of greater than 1 mm in magnitude measured 0.08 s after the J point and persisting for more than 1 min. Significant ST segment elevation was defined as an upward shift of the ST segment of greater than 1 mm in magnitude at the J point compared to the rest of the recording. Changes in the T-wave vector were not regarded as evidence of myocardial ischemia unless they were accompanied by significant ST segment changes.

During all periods of ambulatory monitoring patients kept a detailed diary and pressed an event marker at the onset of symptoms. All patients were encouraged to continue their normal activities during the period of monitoring.

All ischemic episodes in the total duration were categorized on an hourly basis in order to allow a detailed assessment of the frequency distribution of episodes throughout the day. Frequency histograms were produced for all ischemic episodes occurring in the 150 patients off therapy, the patients receiving nifedipine (N = 33) both off and on therapy, and those receiving atenol (N = 41) both off and on therapy.

Statistical analysis

The hourly frequency and durations of total and silent ischemia were subject to Fourier analysis. The optimum number of fitted harmonics was determined as the last harmonic whose addition resulted in a statistically significant reduction in absolute residual squares error. This was found to be a two harmonic fit. Also the 24-h period was divided into four six-h periods and a Chi square test with Yates correction for continuity was applied to determine whether or not there was a significant excess of episodes in the morning hours when compared with the mean of the other three periods. In all cases a P value of less than 0.05 was considered significant.

Results

While the patients were off therapy it was found that episodes of silent ischemia and the total ischemic burden occurred predominantly during the daytime hours from 07.30—19.30 hrs (68 %). There was a significant excess of episodes of total ischemia in the morning hours (07.30—13.30) with a secondary peak occurring in the evening hours.

Thirty-three patients underwent ambulatory ST segment monitoring while receiving nifedipine. A total of 166 episodes of ischemia were recorded while off therapy when the circadian distribution was similar to the group of 150 patients as a whole. On treatment with nifedipine 156 episodes were recorded during 1 313 h of monitoring; 62 (40 %) occurred in the morning hours and 43 (28 %) in the afternoon hours. Again a morning peak in episodes together with a secondary peak was observed as described for the 150 patients off therapy. There was a significant excess of episodes of ischemia occurring in the morning hours. The circadian pattern of the total duration of ischemic episodes closely mimics that of the frequency of episodes with a primary peak of ischemia in the morning hours and a lesser evening peak, both off and on treatment with nifedipine.

Forty-one patients underwent ST segment monitoring while receiving atenolol. A total of 304 episodes were recorded in a subgroup off therapy of which 101 (33 %) occurred in the morning hours and 97 (32 %) in the afternoon hours. In contrast there were 159 episodes of ischemia recorded during 1 581 h of ST segment monitoring when receiving atenolol of which 40 (25 %) occurred in the morning and 55 (35 %) in the afternoon. Off therapy the morning peak in episodes and the secondary evening peak were similar to the findings of the total group. However, when receiving atenolol there is a significant alteration in the circardian pattern of ischemic episodes with elimination of the morning peak in episodes but persistence of the evening peak. No significant difference was discerned between the morning hours and the average of the other three six-h periods in terms of frequency of episodes on treatment with atenolol in contrast to treatment with nifedipine and off therapy. The circadian pattern of total duration of ischemic episodes again closely resembled that of the number of episodes of ischemia with elimination of the morning peak on treatment with atenolol. In addition it was found that atenolol significantly reduced the mean heart rate in all four six-h periods indicating a persistence of beta blockade at the time when evening peak of episodes was occurring.

Discussion

The demonstration that there is significant circadian pattern of ischemic episodes with a peak in the morning hours is of interest. The circadian pattern corresponds closely with the circadian variation recorded for hemodynamic indices (heart rate and blood pressure [1], indices of coagulation [8], catecholamine release [9], and the onset of acute myocardial infarction [3] and sudden death [2].

While there is no direct evidence to suggest a casual relationship between the development of ischemia and acute myocardial infarction and sudden cardiac death it seems reasonable to suggest that they may be inter-related. It is known that sudden cardiac death usually occurs in individuals with severe coronary atherosclerosis and myocardial damage and that patients resuscitated from out of hospital ventricular fibrillation have been shown to have frequent episodes of silent ischemia on exercise testing [4]. We found a similar circadian pattern in the distribution of ischemic episodes to the reported distribution of acute myocardial infarction and sudden death. Pathophysiological and therapeutic implications of this association remain to be explored.

Nifedipine had little effect in altering this circadian distribution of ischemic episodes. Interestingly, Willich has shown that the circadian pattern of acute myocardial infarction is unaltered by calcium antagonists [10]. Atenolol significantly altered the circadian distribution of ischemic episodes, with elimination of the morning peak. This is of interest as Muller has reported that in patients receiving beta blocking agents there was no detectable circadian rhythm of acute myocardial infarction; this finding has been confirmed by Willich et al. [2, 10]. Atenolol appeared to be somewhat less effective in reducing the frequency of ischemic episodes in the evening hours despite a similar reduction in heart rate at the onset of ischemia. This period corresponded with a lesser peak in ischemic episodes which was detected in all groups studied. It is noteworthy that in the beta blocker heart attack trial propranolol resulted in a significant overall reduction in sudden cardiac death, however the reduction occurred between 0200 and 1400 hrs; there was an 18 % increase of sudden cardiac death when compared with placebo from 1400 to 0200 hrs [10]. Again it would appear that there is an association between the circadian distribution of ischemia and the reported distribution of acute myocardial infarction and sudden death even when this distribution is altered by beta blocking drugs.

These studies do not in any way suggest a cause and effect relationship between silent ischemia and sudden cardiac death and acute myocardial infarction. Nor does the fact that nifedipine did not alter the circadian distribution have any implication in terms of the efficacy of this drug in the treatment and prevention of sudden cardiac death and acute myocardial infarction. However, the similarity of patterns of the circadian distribution of silent ischemia and the important end points of coronary disease is of interest and requires further investigation.

References

1. Miller-Craig MW, Bishop CN, Raftery EB (1978) Circadian variation of blood pressure. Lancet 1: 795—797
2. Muller JE, Stone PH, Turi ZG, et al. (1985) Circadian variation in the frequency of onset of acute myocardial infarction. New Eng J Med 313: 1315—1322
3. Muller JE, Ludmer PL, Willich SN, et al. (1987) Circadian variation in the incidence of sudden cardiac death in the Framingham Heart Study population. Am J Cardiol 60: 801—806
4. Perper JA, Kuller LH, Cooper M (1975) Arteriosclerosis of coronary arteries in sudden, unexpected deaths. Circulation 51/52 (Suppl 111): 111—127
5. Peters R, Muller JE, Goldstein S, Byington R, Friedman LM (1987) Propranolol and the circadian variation in the frequency of sudden cardiac death: the BHAT experience. Circulation 76 (Suppl IV): 364 (Abst.)
6. Rocco MB, Barry J, Cambell S, et al. (1987) Circadian variation of transient myocardial ischemia in patients with coronary artery disease. Circulation 75: 395—400
7. Selwyn AP, Shea M, Deanfield JE, Wilson R, Horlock P, O'Brien HA (1986) Character of silent ischemia in angina pectoris. Am J Cardiol 58: 21B—25B
8. Tofler GH, Brezinski D, Schafer AI, et al (1987) Concurrent morning increase in platelet aggregability and the risk of myocardial infarction and sudden death. New Eng J Med 316: 1514—1518
9. Turton NB, Deggan T (1974) Circadian variations of plasma catecholamine, cortisol, and immunoreactive insulin concentrations in supine subjects. Clin Chim Acta 55: 389—397
10. Willich SN, Linderer T, Wegscheider K, Schroder R (1988) Increased risk of myocardial infarction in the morning. J Am Coll Cardiol 11: 28A (Abst.)

Authors' address:
Kim Fox
National Heart Hospital
Westmoreland Street
London W 1, UK

Discussion

KRUCOFF:

Were any of the patients subgroups you discussed on aspirin or other platelet inhibitor therapy and have you looked at that and its relationship to this circadian pattern?

FOX:

No, it would not be possible to do such a study because there is an epidemic use of aspirin in the United Kingdom, whether it is prescribed by the doctor or not. But at the time when we were doing those studies none of the patients were taking aspirin and clearly aspirin would be very interesting, perhaps more in the unstable situation and the timing of ischemic events in unstable angina than chronic stable angina, but that is just hypothesis and that would certainly be very intersting to look at. There have been data on the effects of aspirin in patients with variant angina and it appeared that aspirin had little effect on either the number or the timing of ischemic episodes.

VON ARNIM:

What were your dosing regimes for nifedipine and atenolol, because I think that might have an effect also because you dose your drugs more during the daytime and more in the morning, or did you do a single-dose regimen?

FOX:

The dosing regimen of atenolol was 100 milligrams once a day in the morning. That is why it appears to show a heart rate effect still in the evening. For the dosing regimen of nifedipine we follow a standard regimen for all our studies and that is to use 10 milligrams TDS, followed by 20 milligrams TDS. So some of the patients would have been on 10 milligrams TDS, if they were intolerant of the dose of 20 milligrams TDS.

LEMMER:

There is abolition of the morning peak with beta-blocker as well as with combined treatment of beta-blockers and calcium antagonists. Could not this indicate that beta receptor mediated effects predominate at this time of the day and not at other times of the day? Alpha receptor mediated effects could predominate at late afternoon or morning hours; I think we must look at different systems at different times of day.

FOX:

That is absolutely right. There is a catecholamine surge in the morning and one might expect the beta-blockers to block that.

SIEGRIST:

It would be interesting to know whether a certain portion of your patients were back at work on the treatment and it would be nice to see whether those exposed to working conditions differ in their circadian pattern also on the pharmacotherapy.

FOX:

These studies were performed with patients during their normal daily activities: I do not have data comparing, particularly, the women who might have been at home against that of the workers, or the manual workers vs the non-manual workers. Nor unfortunately do I have any shift workers in that group, although it would have been intersting to repeat the data in those particular patients.

HUBER:

Which drug is able to suppress the evening peak of myocardial events?

FOX:

I can not answer that because we have not investigated sufficient numbers of drugs, one needs to try looking at this with the relative drugs. It is quite hard work, however, because you need at least 30 or 40 patients to describe the statistics for the morning and the evening peaks.

MASERI:

There is a hidden problem in studying circadian variation, one that you did mention: you need large numbers. If you need a large number of patients then one should be very careful in selecting patients that represent the most homogenous population. I am impressed by the varieties of behavior of different patients, which may reflect a different prevelance of pathogenetic mechanisms. By taking large numbers of patients, if one finds a certain pattern, it means that this pattern is very prevalent in that group, but not necessarily all the patients will have the same sort of pattern and therefore not necessarily all the patients may have the prevalence of a given pathogenetic mechanism.

FOX:

You are absolutely right. Even studying only one patient would not help, because I don't believe that one patient will have the same pathogenetic mechanism over the 24-h period: Different mechanisms will be operating even within the same patients, so the point you raise is absolutely correct.
We are looking at the most prevalent mechanisms in a type of patient that are referred to our kind of institution, that is, people with severe three-vessel disease, usually with low exercise tolerance, but again, even within individual patients, I think there will be a variation in the pathogenetic mechanisms causing their angina.

MATHES:

From a previous experience we always tend to associate an accent of changes in vasomotor tone with silent ischemia; from your data, however, one would guess that abolition of the sympathetic drive would really be all that is required to evade the danger of silent ischemia, although beta blockade really increases vasomotor tone just by leaving the alpha receptors open to the sympathetic drive.

FOX:

I think the consensus is beginning to swing away from the concept that silent ischemia is due to a different mechanism than that of angina pectoris. I think the mechanisms causing angina pectoris will include myocardial oxygen demand, will include vasomotor tone, and will probably in the majority of patients include a combination. I think the evidence is beginning to accumulate that silent ischemia differs from angina only in that there is no pain and all those mechanisms which are predominant in angina will also be active in silent ischemia. I think the earlier concept, that silent ischemia was a flow problem and angina was a demand problem is not correct and that both are due to multiple mechanisms.

MASERI:

Data have been in the literature for a long time that myocardial infarction can occur without symptoms and that you can have an exercise test which is very positive, but you do not have pain. You cannot mistake 10 mm ST segment elevation in a patient who has variant angina with, for example 1 mm, 2 mm ST segment depression during an exercise test. So that really must mean something, and therefore it became very striking in variant angina. There have been a tremendous number of meetings in which I realize I was invited to talk about silent ischemia, I was talking about silent ischemia in variant angina and then the heading idea was that if you have silent ischemia now you know how you have to treat your patients.

FOX:

At the end of the day drugs that are effective in angina, beta-blockers, calcium antagonists, nitrates are effective in silent ischemia.

MATHES:

Although the mechanisms may be different.

18

FOX:

Sure, but I think the mechanism of the drugs may be different and clearly in some patients a calcium antagonist will be preferable to a beta-blocker and vice versa in different patients and even in the same patients at different times.

DEEG:

You showed a 24-h circadian rhythm, but what about a weekly or a monthly circadian rhythm?

FOX:

There will certainly be a monthly circadian rhythm in our country. Undoubtedly, we just need to speak to patients to know that the kind of patients we are looking at will be worse in the winter months and painful ischemia will certainly be more frequent. Although we have not looked at silent ischemia in the winter months as opposed to summer months, I guess there will be a difference. The same with variant angina, there will be a daily variation depending on various circumstances. whether some patients are in a hot phase or a cold phase. So there are weekly, monthly, daily rhythms within individual patients.

MASERI:

In Pisa we were seeing, before the widespread use of calcium antagonists, a large number of patients with variant angina with a large number of episodes. What we noticed is that there was some sort of two-week pattern, with peaks every two weeks. But it is really difficult to find a circadian pattern: if you want to have a longer circadian pattern it becomes even more difficult, because you need a larger number of episodes, you need a larger number of patients who are more or less in the same phase of the disease over a long time. This is very unlikely because the disease tends either to get worse and become a myocardial infarction or to get better and this works spontaneously.

KRUCOFF:

I would like to push one step further in terms of our lack of understanding about mechanism and even application of drug classes relative to the markers of their efficacy that we measure. I think it may well be that as we look, for instance, at the impact on circadian variation by beta blockers or calcium blockers that we find that there are both beta and calcium blockers that have antiplatelet effects and other beta and calcium blockers that do not.

Inhibition of fibrinolysis in blood: circadian fluctuation and possible relevance to coronary artery disease

F. Andreotti*, G. J. Davies*, A. Maseri*, and C. Kluft+

* Cardiovascular Research Unit RPMS, Hammersmith Hospital, London, UK,
+TNO Gaubius Institute, Leiden, The Netherlands

Introduction

The end-product of coagulation is a clot with a fibrin meshwork. Fibrin, however, is not a permanent structure, but stimulates a biochemical pathway that leads to its lysis pathway and fragmentation of the clot. Essential components of this, as a consequence, are the plasminogen activators (PAs). PAs convert the zymogen plasminogen to the ultimate fibrinolytic enzyme plasmin (Fig. 1). At least two types of PAs have been identified in plasma: one produced and secreted by endothelial cells (first isolated in urine), called tissue-type PA (t-PA), and another called urinary-type PA or urokinase (UK). UK was later also identified in plasma, mainly as a proenzyme known as pro-urokinase (pro-UK). t-PA and pro-UK both activate plasminogen, preferentially in the presence of fibrin, but by different mechanisms (for review, see [5]).

After clot formation function, the maintenance of fibrin is temporarily ensured by the presence, in excess, of fast-acting, natural inhibitors of fibrinolysis. This inhibition functions at two levels: at the level of formed plasmin, mostly through the action of a-2-antiplasmin, and at the level of plasmin formation, mainly through the action of plasminogen activator inhibitor 1 (PAI-1). The latter neutralizes the two PAs, thereby hindering the conversion of plasminogen to plasmin. In the presence of thrombus, inhibition of fibrinolysis is promoted by the selective binding of a-2-antiplasmin to fibrin and by the local release of large amounts of PAI-1 from platelets. Both a-2-antiplasmin and PAI-1, however, are unstable [31]; PAI-1, in particular, declines rapidly with a half-life at 37 °C of 90 min (for review of PAIs, see [55]).

Inhibitors of fibrinolysis, therefore, contribute to the hemostatic process by initially stabilizing fibrin; the subsequent decline of their activity allows fibrin to lyze. It is conceivable that increased inhibition of fibrinolysis during the initial phase of clot formation may prolong the life-span of fibrin deposits and contribute to the development of a substantial thrombus. The role of PAI-1 in clot survival has been illustrated by in vitro experiments showing delayed lysis of blood clots obtained from subjects with a high level of circulating PAI-1 [8]. PAI-1 is produced by hepatocytes, endothelial cells and, presumably, megakaryocytes, hepatocytes. t-PA and PAI-1 are major determinants of the so-called spontaneous fibrinolytic activity of blood.

The advent of assays for the activity and antigen levels of individual components of the fibrinolytic system have made the assessment of blood fibrinolytic activity

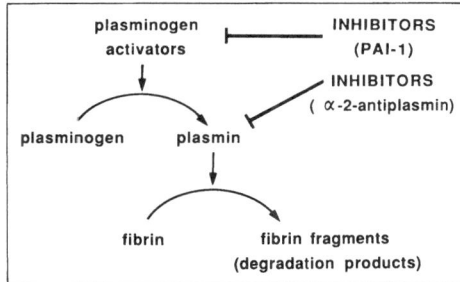

Fig. 1. Scheme of the fibrinolytic cascade.

(BFA) more sensitive and specific. This should be kept in mind when interpreting earlier data based on global methods, such as clot lysis time or fibrin plate lysis area.

Fibrinolysis and atherosclerosis

Ever since Rokitansky in the 1840s conceived the theory of fibrin deposition on the arterial intima as the primary lesion in atherosclerosis, investigators have been anxions to establish whether a defect in the fibrinolytic system might play a role in the development of atheroma.

Several investigators have measured fibrinolytic parameters in blood samples of patients with atherosclerosis. It may be worth noting that most patients in these studies had not had a documented thrombotic event. One early study failed to demonstrate a reduction of basal blood fibrinolytic activity (BFA) in atherosclerotic patients [42]. A subsequent study performed to determine the effects of age, hypertriglyceridemia, or atherosclerotic coronary disease on fibrinolysis confirmed a normal fibrinolytic activity in blood samples taken in the early morning, but showed a reduction in the physiologic diurnal increment of fibrinolytic activity in relation to all three of the above parameters [52]. Also, in 25 patients with angiographically documented coronary atherosclerosis a reduced local accumulation of t-PA in response to the venous occlusion test was observed, compared to subjects with normal coronary arteriograms [61].

More recently, plasma levels of PAI activity and of t-PA-related antigen were found to be significantly higher in 118 patients with different degrees of angiographically assessed coronary stenoses, compared to apparently healthy, age-matched controls. There was, however, no correlation between the level of fibrinolytic factors and the degree of coronary lesions [48]. Another study confirmed the lack of correlation between the degree of coronary atherosclerosis and PAI activity levels; furthermore, in this study, elevated PAI activity in patients, compared to a younger control group, was attributed to the effect of age [40]. The latter is in agreement with the reported physiologic increase of PAI-1 in relation to age [1, 24, 35]. One further study has reported increased PAI activity in patients with coronary atherosclerotic disease, compared to younger controls [35].

These data seem to indicate that early morning basal BFA may not be altered in atherosclerotic subjects, whereas the diurnal variation and the response to venous occlusion may be impaired. The latest data on specific fibrinolytic factors suggest that elevated blood levels of PAI-1 may in fact be normal for age; this, however, needs careful verification. Several reports on increased t-PA antigen levels in relation to age should also be considered [1, 50]. In addition to the effect of age, future studies should take into account the pronounced diurnal variations of t-PA and PAI-1. Ultimately, it will be necessary to determine to what extent abnormalities of fibrinolytic parameters in atherosclersis are of etiological significance rather than a simple association or a secondary phenomenon.

Fibrinolysis and myocardial infarction

To establish the role of fibrinolytic abnormalities in the development of arterial thrombosis, in vitro and clinical studies have examined conditions directly related to the presence of a thrombus. After the definitive establishment of the causal role of thrombi in myocardial infarction (MI) [13], several studies have concentrated on controlled groups of patients with MI.

Transient changes in blood fibrinolytic activity (BFA) have been identified in the acute phase of MI. In the first 6—8 hrs (hyper-acute phase) a short-lived rise in BFA seems to occur [47, 34], which appears related to t-PA [54]. In the following period (12 h—1 week), there is a marked drop in BFA which is maximal within 48 h and lasts 8—10 days [26, 47, 18]. Recent studies have identified PAI-1 as the main factor responsible for this transient reduction in BFA [29, 19, 2].

Although these changes support the involvement of the fibrinolytic system in the early phases of infarction, they seem to reflect more a response to myocardial injury than a cause of intravascular thrombosis. Indeed, the initial increase in t-PA activity resembles other well-known stress-induced increases in t-PA, such as those observed during the early intra-operative period [56], whereas the later increase in PAI-1 may be an aspecific acute-phase response of PAI-1 to tissue injury [29, 36].

Stronger support for the involvement of fibrinolytic factors in the etiology of coronary thrombosis can be derived from several large-scale studies in patients with previous MI, which have consistently detected an alteration in fibrinolysis [9, 17, 21, 22, 46]. The most recent of these studies, as well as some smaller-scale ones [15, 60], have shown that the abnormality consists of increased levels of PAI-1, and this increase appears to be greater in relatively young patients [21, 22], in the presence of hypertriglyceridemia [21, 46, 40], and in patients with a previous MI but with angiographically normal coronary arteries [60]. A correlation has also been reported between plasma levels of fibrinolytic factors (reduced t-PA activity or increased PAI activity) and the risk of reinfarction [19, 23].

Circadian rhythms and thrombotic tendency

Over the last decade a number of investigations based on epidemiologic data have convincingly shown that clinical events associated with occlusive arterial thrombosis, such as acute MI [13], sudden cardiac death [12] and stroke [37], occur more frequently in the morning. The time of highest incidence is 9.00—10.00 hours for both acute MI [43, 64] and sudden cardiac death [44, 62], and between 24.00 and 6.00 hours for stroke [39].

It is tempting, from these observations, to speculate on possible circadian changes in the hemostatic balance and, indeed, several studies have investigated this aspect. A frequent (every 3 h) assessment over 24 h in normal subjects showed a significant circadian variation in PTT (shortest at 03.00 hours), as well as in thrombin time (TT) and Howell's time (both shortest at 09.00 hours) [49]. Platelet aggregation with ADP was also measured and found to be significantly higher at 12.00 hours. Interestingly, a group of age-matched atherosclerotic patients showed no circadian variation of Howell's time or platelet aggregation and a different pattern, consistent with a delay of 3 h, of the circadian values of PTT and TT [49].

A recent study in normal subjects on circadian platelet aggregation in response to ADP and epinephrine reported increased aggregability between 06.00 and 09.00 hours, coinciding with the assumption of upright posture and with increased plasma catecholamines. In a control group confined to morning bedrest, platelet aggregability and catecholamine levels did not exhibit this morning increase [57]. The authors suggest that activation of the sympathetic nervous system may be responsible for the changes in platelet aggregability. Similar results have been reported for patients with coronary artery disease [63]. On the other hand, an earlier study on circadian platelet adhesiveness in normals showed highest values at 24.00 hours and lowest values between 07.00 and 09.00 hours [10].

The scarce information on circadian levels of circulating anticoagulants concerns the activity of antithrombin III, which showed no circadian variation in normal subjects, but a significant decrease at 06.00 hours in age-matched atherosclerotic patients [49].

Although not conclusive, these data suggest that a state of relative thrombophilia may be present between 24.00 hours and 12.00 hours, compared to the rest of the 24-h cycle.

Circadian and diurnal variations of fibrinolysis

Several reports, early and recent, have demonstrated a circadian variation in basal blood fibrinolytic activity (BFA). The first of these studies, based on dilute blood clot lysis time, recorded in normal subjects a sinusoidal fluctuation of BFA over 24 h, with peak activity at 18.00 hours and nadir at 04.00 hours [16]. Very similar results were later reported [10, 53]. Other studies confirmed the existence of a diurnal increase in BFA, between 08.00 hours and 16.00 hours [38, 41, 51]. Reduced circadian levels of BFA have been observed in patients with severe hypertriglyceridemia, compared to well-matched controls [53], and in association with ischemic heart disease [11].

In the last decade, assays for measuring individual components of the fibrinolytic system have become available. Diurnal changes of t-PA activity were first reported in 1978, with a two-to-threefold increase between 09.00 hours and 15.00 hours [28]. Later, the activity of the fast inhibitor of t-PA, PAI-1, was found to exhibit an opposite pattern, with a twofold drop from 09.00 hours to 15.00 hours. Levels of t-PA antigen, representing both free t-PA and inhibitor-complexed t-PA, also showed a significant drop of about 20—30 % from morning to early afternoon [30, 45]. Recently, the plasma levels of PAI-1 antigen have been measured and also found to decrease significantly from 09.00 hours to 15.00 hours, while the activity of a reversible inhibitor of t-PA does not vary [32].

The divergence in the diurnal changes of t-PA activity (increase) and of t-PA antigen (decrease) has been attributed to the inhibitory effect of PAI-1 on t-PA activity [32]. The concordance in the diurnal changes of t-PA and PAI-1 antigens (both decreased) has suggested a co-ordinated and fluctuating production of these two proteins by endothelial cells [32]. This concept is further supported by the finding of structural homologies in the genomic code of both proteins [7]. In a 12-h study (from 08.00 hours to 20.00 hours), the diurnal increase of BFA was also found to be determined by a decline in PAI-1 antigen levels rather than by an increase in the levels of t-PA or UK antigens [20].

Circadian fluctuation of fibrinolytic factors in normals and in atherosclerotic patients

In order to interpret correctly the data on fibrinolytic factors based on blood samples taken at a fixed time of day, it is necessary to know beforehand whether the circadian pattern is altered. Little information exists on the complete circadian pattern of fibrinolytic components, both in normals or in disease states.

We have investigated this aspect in six healthy subjects (four men and two women, mean 28 years), one "apparently normal" volunteer (female, 26 years) and six atherosclerotic patients (all male, mean 64 years). The six healthy subjects were non-smokers, normolipidemic, took no drugs or oral contraceptives, and performed usual daily activities. These subjects were considered to be relatively free from atherosclerosis and served as controls. The "apparently normal" volunteer did not differ from the control group except for the use of oral contraceptives (OC). The atherosclerotic patients were hospitalized for clinically and angiographically severe disease affecting the aorta and the peripheral or carotid arteries; two patients also had documented coronary artery disease.

Blood samples were taken every 3 h for 24 h (from 09.00 hours until 09.00 hours the next morning) through an indwelling peripheral venous cannula, into pre-cooled, citrated plastic tubes, and immediately centrifuged at 4 °C. Aliquots of platelet-poor plasma were snap-frozen within 1 h of collection and stored at −70 °C.

t-PA activity was determined in plasma euglobulin fractions by the parabolic rate assay described by Verheijen [58] and expressed in milli-International Units per ml (mIU/ml). Plasma PAI-activity was determined by titration with purified t-PA and expressed as percentage of a reference pooled plasma (standard 290385 shown to neutralize 7.6 IU t-PA/ml) [58]. t-PA antigen was determined by enzyme immunoassay (Imulyse t-PA Biopool AB, Umea, Sweden). Total UK antigen was determined by enzyme immunoassay using purified goat anti-UK IgG [6]. The inactive pro-urokinase (pro-UK) and the active UK antigens were determined by bioimmunoassay, before and after activation of pro-UK with plasmin [14]. The UK-inhibitor complex (UK-Inh) was calculated by subtracting the antigen concentration of both pro-UK and active UK from that of total UK. Antigen concentrations in plasma are expressed in ng/ml. Mean peak and nadir values were compared by Student's *t*-tests.

Results and discussion

We previously documented the physiologic variation of individual components of the fibrinolytic system over a 24-h period in normal subjects [3, 4]. Figures 2 and 3 exemplify these results. As can be noted, not all factors showed the same degree of variation. For t-PA antigen, t-PA activity and PAI activity (Fig. 2), a highly significant difference between peak and nadir values was observed in all three parameters

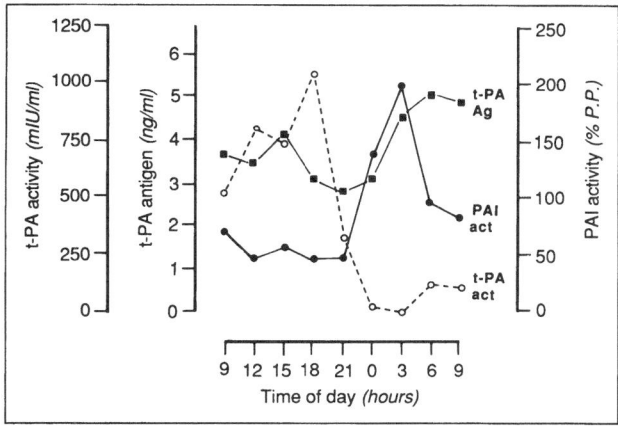

Fig. 2. Circadian plasma levels of t-PA and PAI activities and t-PA antigen in a typical, normal subject

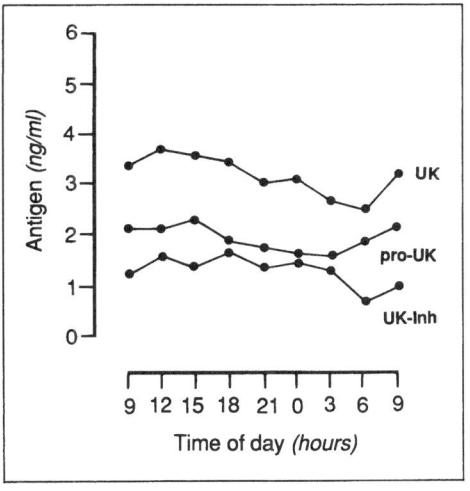

Fig. 3. Circadian plasma levels of total urokinase (UK), pro-urokinase, and UK-inhibitor complex (same subject as in Fig. 2)

25

(p < 0.01). For components of the urokinase system, on the other hand, minor changes (p < 0.05) were recorded only in pro-urokinase and UK-inhibitor complex (Fig. 3). Furthermore, for t-PA and PAI-1, the times of peaks and nadirs showed greater inter-individual consistency than for the urokinase-related factors (individual curves not shown).

The circadian fluctuation of t-PA activity closely resembles the known circadian rhythm of fibrinolysis assessed with global methods; this lends additional support to the concept that t-PA activity is a major determinant of overall fibrinolytic activity in blood. The temporal coincidence between peak t-PA activity and lowest PAI activity at 18.00 hours and between peak PAI and lowest t-PA activities at 03.00 hours suggests a strong inverse relation between these two factors. In contrast, t-PA antigen and t-PA activity do not show a close temporal relation, with an interval of 9—12 h between their peaks.

Theoretically, increased PAI activity may result from a rise in PAI-1 antigen or a drop in t-PA or UK antigens. The observed increase of PAI activity during the night cannot be explained by changes in t-PA or UK antigen levels at that time, since t-PA antigen increased and UK antigen remained constant. This suggests that the level of PAI-1 antigen is the major determinant of the circadian changes in both t-PA and PAI activities.

Table 1 summarizes and compares the results of circadian t-PA and PAI activities, and t-PA antigen in normal and atherosclerotic patients. In both, normals and patients, t-PA and PAI activities showed a significant circadian variation. The mean 24-h level of t-PA activity was lower in the patient group, but this difference did not reach statistical significance. Interestingly, the timing of peak and nadir t-PA and PAI activities showed a 3-h delay in the atherosclerotic subjects. The patients' concentration of t-PA antigen was strikingly higher, compared to normals, but the amplitude and phase of the fluctuation were similar in the two groups. Such high t-PA antigen levels may reflect an increase in t-PA production by endothelium or a reduction in t-PA clearance by the liver. The combination of elevated t-PA antigen levels with normal or reduced t-PA activity in patients suggests an increase in circulating t-PA-inhibitor complexes.

Levels of t-PA and PAI-1, in blood samples taken in the early morning, are significantly altered by anabolic steroids [59] and oral contraceptives (OC) [27]. It is

Table 1: Circadian levels (mean ± SD) of t-PA and PAI activities, and t-PA antigen in normal and in atherosclerotic patients (ATS).

	t-PA activity (mIU/ml)		PAI activity (% P.P.)		t-PA antigen (ng/ml)	
	Normal	ATS	Normal	ATS	Normal	ATS
Peak value	779±390	410±352	193±60	186±50	7.1±1.3	18±53
Time of peak	18.00	21.00	03.00	06.00	09.00	09.00
Nadir value	5±7	6±7	53±14	77±35	4.3±1.8	13.4±4.8
Time of nadir	03.00	06.00	18.00	21.00	24.00	21.00
Peak vs nadir	p<0.005	p<0.05	p<0.001	p<0.05	p<0.01	NS
24 h mean	297±283	113±134	96±47	121±42	5.7±1	15±1.4

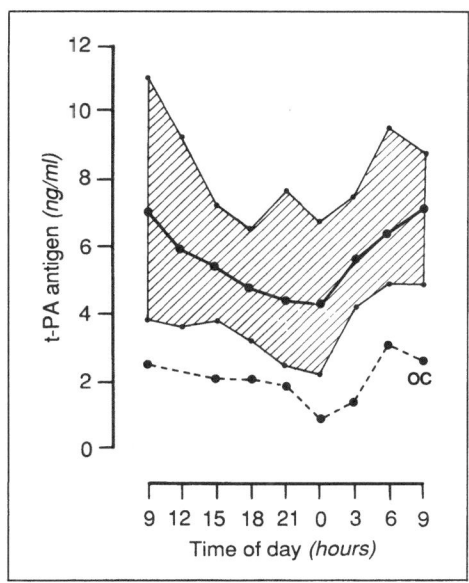

Fig. 4. Circadian pattern of t-PA antigen in a volunteer taking oral contraceptives. The hatched area represents the mean values and total zange in six control subjects

not known, however, in what way these drugs affect the underlying circadian pattern. In the "apparently normal" volunteer using OC, the reported reduction in PAI activity [27] was mantained during the whole 24-h study period (see Table 1 for range in controls). The circadian pattern of t-PA antigen in this volunteer is shown in Fig. 4. As for PAI activity, t-PA antigen levels were lower, ranging from 0.9 ng/ml at 24.00 hours to 3.1 ng/ml at 06.00 hours; the phase of the circadian rhythm, however, was similar to that seen in the control subjects.

As, recently pointed out [33] and illustrated by these data, it is clear, that changes in t-PA and PAI-1 may result from one or more alterations of the circadian pattern affecting the amplitude of variation, the phase of the sinusoidal fluctuation, or the mean 24-h level. Therefore for an accurate investigation of these factors a 24-h study should be performed [33].

Conclusion

Among the various parameters involved in hemostasis, blood fibrinolytic activity (BFA) shows the most striking and well-documented circadian variation. Variation in spontaneous BFA is regulated predominantly by fibrinolytic inhibitors, particularly PAI-1. The marked increase of PAI activity during the early morning hours may contribute to the higher morning incidence of arterial thrombotic events.

References

1. Aillaud MF, Pignol F, Alessi MC, Harle JR, Escande M, Mongin M, Juhan-Vague I (1986) Increase in plasma concentration of plasminogen activator inhibitor, fibrinogen, von Willebrand

factor, factor VIII: C and in erythrocyte sedimentation rate with age. Thromb Haemost 55: 330—332

2. Almer L-O, Ohlin H (1987) Elevated levels of the rapid inhibitor of plasminogen-activator (t-PAI) in acute myocardial infarction. Thromb Res 47: 335—339
3. Andreotti F, Davies GJ, Hackett D, Khan MI, deBart A, Aber VR, Maseri A, Kluft C (1988) Major circadian fluctuations of fibrinolytic factors and possible relevance to time of onset of myocardial infarction, sudden cardiac death and stroke. Am J Cardiol, in press.
4. Andreotti F, Davies GJ, Hackett D, Khan MI, deBart A, Dooijewaard G, Maseri A, Kluft C (1988) Circadian variation of fibrinolytic factors in normal human plasma. Fibrinolysis 2 (2): 90—92
5. Bachmann F (1987) Fibrinolysis. In: Verstraete M, Vermylen J, Leijnen L, Arnout J (eds) Thrombosis and Haemostasis. and Leuven University Press, Leuven, p 227—265
6. Binnema DJ, van Iersel JJL, Dooijewaard G (1986) Quantitation of urokinase antigen in plasma and culture media by use of an ELISA. Thromb Res 43: 569—577
7. Bosma PJ, van den Berg EA, Kooistra T, Siemieniak DR, Slightom JL (1988) Human plasminogen activator inhibitor-1 gene; promoter and structural gene nucleotide sequences. J Biol Chem in press
8. Brommer EJP, Boks AL, Koopman J, Haverkate F (1985) Protraction of whole blood and plasma clot lysis in patients with high levels of an inhibitor of tissue-type plasminogen activator. Thromb Res 39: 271—280
9. Chakrabarti R, Hocking ED, Fearnley GR, Mann RD, Attwell TN, Jackson D (1968) Fibrinolytic activity and coronary artery disease. Lancet 1: 987—990
10. Cepelak VV, Barcal R, Lang N, Cepelakova H (1966) Zum Tag- und Nachtrhythmus der Fibrinolyse. Zschr Inn Med 21: 202—204
11. Cepelak VV, Barcal R, Cepelakova H, Mayer O (1978) Circadian Rhythm of Fibrinolysis In: Davidson JF, Rowan RM, Samama MM, Desnoyers PC, eds. Progress in Chemical Fibrinolysis and Thrombolysis. Raven Press, New York, p 571—578
12. Davies MJ, Thomas A (1984) Thrombosis and acute coronary artery lesions in sudden cardiac ischemic death. N Engl J Med 310: 1137—1140
13. DeWood MA, Spores J, Notske R, Mouser LT, Burroughs R, Golden MS, Lang T (1980) Prevalence of total coronary occlusion during the early hours of transmural myocardial infarction. N Engl J Med 303: 897—902
14. Dooijewaard G, van Iersel JJL, Brommer EJP (1986) Quantitation of Pro-UK, UK and UK. Inhibitor levels in plasma of patients and healthy men. Fibrinolysis 1 (1): A142
15. Estelles A, Tormo G, Aznar J, Espana F, Tormo V (1985) Reduced fibrinolytic activity in coronary heart disease in basal conditions and after exercise. Thromb Res 40: 373—383
16. Fearnley GR, Balmforth G, Fearnley E (1957) Evidence of a diurnal fibrinolytic rhythm; with a simple method of measuring natural fibrinolysis. Clin Sci 16: 645—650
17. Franzen J, Nilsson B, Johansson BW, Nilsson IM (1983) Fibrinolytic activity in men with acute myocardial infarction before 60 years of age. Acta Med Scand 214: 339—344
18. Gidron E, Margalit R, Oliven A, Shalitin Y (1977) Effect of myocardial infarction on components of fibrinolytic system. Br Heart J 39: 19—24
19. Gram J, Jespersen J (1987) A selective depression of tissue plasminogen activator (t-PA) activity in euglobulins characterises a risk group among survivors of acute myocardial infarction. Thromb Haemost 57: 137—139
20. Grimaudo V, Hauert J, Bachmann F, Kruithof EKO (1988) Diurnal variation of the fibrinolytic system. Thromb Haemost 59: 495—499
21. Hamsten A, Wiman B, de Faire U, Blomback M (1985) Increased plasma levels of a rapid inhibitor of tissue plasminogen activator in young survivors of myocardial infarction. N Engl J Med 313: 1557—1563
22. Hamsten A, Blomback M, Wiman B, Svensson J, Szamosi A, de Faire U, Mettinger L (1986) Haemostatic function in myocardial infarction. Br Heart J 55: 58—66
23. Hamsten A, Walldius G, Szamosi A, Blomback M, de Faire U, Dahlen G, Landou C, Wiman B (1987) Plasminogen activator inhibitor in plasma: risk factor for recurrent myocardial infarction. Lancet 2: 3—9
24. Hashimoto T, Kobayashi A, Yamaxaki N, Sugawara Y, Takada Y, Takada A (1987) Relationship between age and plasma t-PA, PA-inhibitor and PA activity. Thromb Res 46: 625

25. Huber K, Resch I, Rose D, Schuster E, Glogar D, Binder BR (1987) Circadian variation of plasminogen activator inhibitor (PAI) and the incidence of severe ischaemic attacks in patients with coronary artery disease. Thromb Haemost 58 (1): A224

26. Hume R (1958) Fibrinolysis in myocardial infarction. Br Heart J 20: 15—20

27. Jespersen J, Kluft C (1986) Inhibition of tissue-type plasminogen activator in women using oral contraceptives and in normal women during a menstrual cycle. Thromb Haemost 55: 388—389

28. Kluft C (1978) Cl-inactivator-resistant fibrinolytic activity in plasma euglobulin fractions: Its relation to vascular activator in blood and its role in euglobulin fibrinolysis. Thromb Res 13: 135—151

29. Kluft C, Verheijen JH, Jie AFH, Rijken DC, Preston FE, Sue-Ling HM, Jespersen J, Aasen AO (1985) The postoperative fibrinolytic shutdown: a rapidly reverting acute phase pattern for the fast-acting inhibitor of tissue-type plasminogen activator after trauma. Scand J Clin Lab Invest 45: 605—610

30. Kluft C, Verheijen JH, Rijken DC, Chang GTG, Jie AFH, Onkelinx C (1985) Diurnal fluctuations in the activity of the fast-acting t-PA inhibitor. In: Davidson JF, Donati MB, Coccheri S (eds) Progress in Fibrinolysis. Churchill-Livingstone, Edinburgh, vol 7, p 117—119

31. Kluft C (1988) t-PA in fibrin dissolution and haemostasis. In: Kluft C (ed) Tissue-type plasminogen activator (t-PA): physiological and clinical aspects. CRC press, Boca Raton, vol 1, p 47—49

32. Kluft C, Jie AFH, Rijken DC, Verheijen JH (1988) Daytime fluctuations in blood of tissue-type plasminogen activator (t-PA) and its fast-acting inhibitor (PAI-1). Thromb Haemost 59: 329—332

33. Kluft C, Andreotti F (1988) Consequences of the circadian fluctuation in plasminogen activator inhibitor 1 (PAI-1) for studies on blood fibrinolysis. Fibrinolysis 2 (2): 93—95

34. Komamura K, Hirayama A, Yamamoto K, Nanto S, Mishima M, Kodoma K (1988) Transient increase in endogenous plasma tissue plasminogen activator in patients with acute myocardial infarction. JACC 11(2): 53A

35. Kruithof EKO, Nicoloso G, Bachmann F (1987) Plasminogen activator inhibitor 1. Development of a radioimmunoassay and observations on its plasma concentration during venous occlusion and after platelet aggregation. Blood 70: 1645—1653

36. Kruithof EKO, Gudinchet A, Bachmann F (1988) PAI-1 and PAI-2 in various disease states. Thromb Haemost 59: 7—12

37. Kunitz SC, Gross CR, Heyman A, Kase CS, Mohr JP, Price TR, Wolf PA (1984) The pilot stroke data bank: definition, design and data. Stroke 15: 740—746

38. Mann RD (1967) Effect of age, sex and diurnal variation on the human fibrinolytic system. J Clin Path 20: 223—226

39. Marshall J (1977) Diurnal variation in occurrence of strokes. Stroke 88: 230—231

40. Mehta J, Mehta P, Lawson D, Saldeen T (1987) Plasma tissue plasminogen activator inhibitor levels in coronary artery disease: correlation with age and serum triglyceride concentrations. JACC 9: 263—268

41. Menon IS, White RWB, Smith PA, Dewar HA (1967) Diurnal variations of fibrinolytic activity and plasma-11-hydroxycorticosteroid levels. Lancet 2: 531—533

42. Merskey C, Gordon H, Lackner H (1960) Blood coagulation and fibrinolysis in relation to coronary heart disease. Br Med J: 219—226

43. Muller JE, Stone PH, Turl ZG, Rutherford JD, Czeisler CA, Parker C, Poole WK et al. (1985) Circadian variation in the frequency of onset of acute myocardial infarction. N Engl J Med 313: 1315—1322

44. Muller JE, Ludmer PL, Willich SN, Tofler GH, Aylmer G, Klangos I, Stone PH (1987) Circadian variation in the frequency of sudden cardiac death. Circulation 75: 131—138

45. Neerstrand H, Ostergaard P, Bergqvist D, Matzsch T, Hedner MU (1987) tPA inhibitor, tPA:Ag, Plasminogen, and α2-antiplasmin after low molecular weight heparin or standard heparin. Fibrinolysis 1: 39—43

46. Nilsson TK, Johnson O (1987) The exztrinsic fibrinolytic system in survivors of myocardial infarction. Thromb Res 48: 621—630

47. Ogston D, Fullerton HW (1965) Plasma fibrinolytic activity following recent myocardial and cerebral infarction. Lancet 2: 99—101

48. Paramo JA, Colucci M, Collen D (1985) Plasminogen activator inhibitor in the blood of patients with coronary artery disease. Br Med J 291: 573—574
49. Petralito A, Mangiafico RA, Gibiino S, Cuffari MA, MIano MF, Fiore CE (1982) Daily modifications of plasma fibrinogen, platelets aggregation, Howell's time, PTT, TT, and antithrombin III in normal subjects and in patients with vascular disease. Chronobiologia 9: 195—201
50. Ranby M, Bergsdorf N, Nilsson T, Mellbring G, Winblad B, Bucht G (1986) Age dependence of tissue plasminogen activator concentrations in plasma, as studied by an improved enzyme-linked immunosorbent assay. Clin Chem 32: 2160—2165
51. Rosing DR, Brakman P, Redwood DR, Goldstein RE, Beiser GD, Astrup T, Epstein SE (1970) Blood fibrinolytic activity in man: Diurnal variation and the response to varying intensities of exercise. Circ Res 27: 171—184
52. Rosing DR, Redwood DR, Brakman P, Astrup T, Epstein SE (1973) Impairment of the diurnal fibrinolytic response in man: effects of aging, type IV hyperlipoproteinemia and coronary artery disease. Circ Res 32: 752—758
53. Simpson HCR, Meade TW, Stirling Y, Mann JI, Chakrabarti R, Woolf L (1983) Hypertriglyceridemia and hypercoagulability. Lancet 1: 786—790
54. Six A, Liem MK, Haas FJLM, van Hemel NM, Dooijewaard G, Kluft C (1988) The state of the fibrinolytic system during the early phase of myocardial infarction and unstable angina. Fibrinolysis 2(1): A15
55. Sprengers ED, Kluft C (1987) Plasminogen activator inhibitors. Blood 69: 381—387.
56. Stibbe J, Kluft C, Brommer EP, Gomes M, de Jong DS, Nauta J (1984) Enhanced fibrinolytic activity during cardiopulmonary bypass in open-heart surgery in man is caused by extrinsic (tissue-type) plasminogen activator. Eur J Clin Invest 14: 375—382
57. Tofler GH, Brezinski D, Schafer AI, Czeisler CA, Ruthenford JD, Willich SN, Gleason RE, Williams GH, Muller JE (1987) Concurrent morning increase in platelet aggregability and the risk of myocardial infarction and sudden cardiac death. N Engl J Med 316: 1514—1518
58. Verheijen JH, Chang GTG, Kluft C (1984) Evidence for the occurrence of a fast acting inhibitor for tissue-type plasminogen activator in human plasma. Thromb Haemost 51: 392—395
59. Verheijen JH, Rijken DC, Chang GTG, Preston FE, Kluft C (1984) Modulation of rapid plasminogen activator inhibitor in plasma by stanozolol. Thromb Haemost 51: 396—397
60. Verheugt FWA, ten Cate JW, Sturk A, Imandt L, Verhorst PMJ, van Eenige MJ, Verwey W, Roos JP (1987) Tissue plasminogen activator activity and inhibition in acute myocardial infarction and angiographically normal coronary arteries. Am J Cardiol 59: 1075—1079
61. Walker ID, Davidson JF, Hutton I, Lawrie TDV (1977) Disordered "fibrinolytic potential" in coronary heart disease. Thromb Res 10: 509—520
62. Willich SN, Levy D, Rocco MB, Tofler GH, Stone PH, Muller JE (1987) Circadian variation in the incidence of sudden cardiac death in the Framingham Heart Study Population. Am J Cardiol 60: 801—806
63. Willich SN, Sintonen SP, Bhatia SS, Tofler GH, Shook TL, Muller JE, Williams GH, Stone PH (1988) Morning increase of platelet aggregability in patients with coronary artery disease. JACC 11: 204A
64. World Health Organization Myocardial Infarction Community Registers (1979) In: Public Health in Europe. Regional Office for Europe (WHO), Copenhagen, Vol 5, p 1—232.

Authors' address:
F. Andreotti
Cardiovascular Research Unit
RPMS, Hammersmith Hospital
Ducane Road
London W 12 ONN, UK

Discussion

LEMMER:

What is the differentiation between age-dependent changes in these rhythms and disease-induced changes in these rhythms. My second question is: do you have any indication whether these rhythms are really endogeneous, free-run, or whether they are triggered by certain "Zeitgebers"?

ANDREOTTI:

To answer the first question, the role of age has been investigated only on samples taken at a single time of day, so I do not have data that document the effect of age on the circadian rhythm. To answer the second question on how endogeneous or triggered rhythms may work I will go to a point raised in the previous discussion, that is studies performed in shift workers. For fibrinolytic activities such a study was performed in 1957. In fact, using the methods available at that time for dilute blood clot lysis time.

It was shown that there was a significant and striking circadian variation of fibrinolytic activity superimposable to the curve that we have documented for TPA activity. This was investigated in nurses who worked during the day and the same pattern was observed in nurses on nightshift, demonstrating the sleep-wake pattern was not strong enough to override this circadian rhythm. It also demonstrates that the effective physical exercise is not a major determinant in fibrinolytic activity, which has also been suggested by others because indeed the strenous excercise does increase fibrinolytic activity in blood.

FOX:

One has to be careful with nurses and some shift workers because they change their patterns very quickly and it may take longer than one or two days to reset the mechanisms. Has anyone looked up nurses and shift workers who constantly worked nights?

ANDREOTTI:

I assume they were night workers for a considerable period of time. This transitional period that you allude to has been well documented in animal studies, where you can see day to day shifts of one, two, three hours in patterns for body temperature, for instance.

MATHES:

From your data the lowest peak in inhibitory activity is apparent very early in the morning. That is a difference between this time and the occurence of the highest incidence of infarctions. Would you say this must be a precursor; would you like to speculate on the incidence between infarct and PAI activity?

ANDREOTTI:

I understand that you are referring to the observations where in some subjects the peak of the inhibitor was observed at midnight, or 03.00 hours. In the normal young group there were six subjects, four out of six had a peak at 03.00 hours, one at 24.00 hours, one at 06.00 hours, so that averages to 03.00 hours, which is a bit sooner than the peak incidence of myocardiac infarction, as you say. Interstingly, in the patient group there was this 3-h shift to a later peak at 06.00 hours. It did not reach statistical significance.

To possibly explain that delay you have to consider the dynamics of thrombotic occlusion in the coronary system — there would not be an instant phenomenon; it will be a form of balance and shift towards greater thrombogenicity and higher PAI-1.

MATHES:

Would you regard this as a precursor for the trombus formation?

ANDREOTTI:

Yes, I would, but I would definitely not consider it the main, the only determinant. Increased activation of thrombotic plaques, platelet aggregation, or activation of the sympathetic system, all may contribute to the shift phenomenon.

HUBER:

Are your data from patients who were ambulatory and did normal physical exercise, and do you have data about patients who rested the whole day?

ANDREOTTI:

Patients were hospitalized. Therefore, they differ to a certain extent with the normal group that pursued their normal activities. They were not bed-ridden, however, and they did get up during the day and walked. I do not personally have data on circadian rhythms in patients that were bedridden, others however, have documented this. They observed a blunting in the circadian rhythm in subjects that were bedridden. I have already referred, however, to another study that did not confirm this. In other words, we do not believe that activity is going to basically alter the circadian rhythm of fibrinolytic activity.

LEMMER:

If I remember right, the half-life of these proteins is rather short. Do you have any indication that there will be a change in the half-life with time of day so that the cleavage will be changed?

ANDREOTTI:

That is a possible explanation, that the pharmacodynamics of these drugs in blood may vary over 24 h and your very interesting report substantiates such a concept. We have not documented this.

VON ARNIM:

When one sees your activity curve on TPA and PAI going sort of symmetric, one asks how much the assays may be inter-related or independent and the question is whether you have an assay which would measure the sum of the two, and which one overrides the other? Is there really a rise in overall thrombogenicity in the early morning hours?

ANDREOTTI:

The assays I think are not confined in these results. PAI activity, as in particular, does assess the summation as you say, of both factors in plasma and it is defined as the amount of TPA that you add exogenously in the assay condition that is necessary to neutralize the PAI activity. For given free TPA, which you know is very low, PAI activity still varies in such a manner over the 24 h.

I could go a little further in the assay for TPA activity and specify that we do not take plasma directly to measure TPA activity. It is known that TPA activity in plasma is very low or undetectable, therefore it is necessary to precipitate the plasma protein and test the fractions for TPA. This procedure presumably removes the inhibitor components and enables one to test the actual TPA activity as a reflection of the free circulating TPA activity in blood.

Life-events as precursors of unstable angina pectoris

H. W. Gerbig, Th. von Arnim

Medizinische Klinik I, Klinikum Großhadern, Ludwig Maximilians Universität, Munich, FRG

Introduction

Life event research has focused on the observation of stressful events in context with the onset of various diseases. Life events are individual stressful experiences like severe illness, loss of a partner, or other events that interrupt daily life routine and demand coping activity of the individual. Associations could be shown for example with tuberculosis, hernia inguinalis, pregnancy disturbances, and psychiatric diseases [4, 1, 10, 3, 5]. Some studies demonstrated an association between acute myocardial infarction (AMI) and also sudden cardiac death as well as a cumulation of life events shortly before the beginning of the disease [14, 12, 8, 7, 13, 15, 6].

One of the most frequently cited studies was published by CM. Parkes; its title is "Broken Heart" and he investigated the mortality of widowers and their post mortem pathological findings. The mortality rate of these men in the first six months after the death of their spouses was 40% higher than the rate for married men of the same age. The incidence of CHD as cause of death shows the most marked difference between the groups [6], but other causes of death are also more frequent in the newly widowed.

Siegrist investigated patients with AMI in comparison to a control group without cardiovascular disease, and he showed that the patients with AMI experienced more frequent and more severe life events. These events cumulated before infarction [10].

When life events precede AMI, they also should be precursors of UAP. The aim of our present study was to answer the following questions:
1) Did the patients show more frequent and more severe life events in the two years before the onset of UAP in comparison to patients with stable angina pectoris?
2) Do these events cumulate in the last three months in the group of patients with UAP?

Materials and methods

Twenty-one male patients in our coronary care unit with UAP (group I) were consecutively entered into the study if they fulfilled the following inclusion criteria:
— angina pectoris which shows progression in duration, severity, and frequency, as a change of symptoms of a preexisting stable angina, or a new onset of angina with a progressive character;
— CHD must be proven by coronary angiography.

33

Exclusion criteria were defined as:
— signs of AMI such as irreversible ECG changes or significant increase of creatin kinase;
— age > 80 years or age < 21 years:
— physical or psychological inability to cooperate;
— treatable causes of angina pectoris, like severe anemia, or arrhythmias, or hyperviscosity;
— AMI less than seven days before.

Every patient underwent actual coronary angiography. As controls we selected patients matched pairs for age, sex, and severity of fixed CHD (following the Gensini score [2°], but without unstable symptoms. These 21 matched control patients form group II.

Both groups did not differ significantly in age (mean age 57.9 vs 57.6 years) or in the number of coronary vessels diseased (Fig. 1). Looking at the Gensini score, there was a tendency to a angiographically more severe CHD of group I (UAP). This discrepancy could not be avoided in some matched pairs with severe or extreme extent of CHD, because stable angina was rare in this population. (Mean Gensini

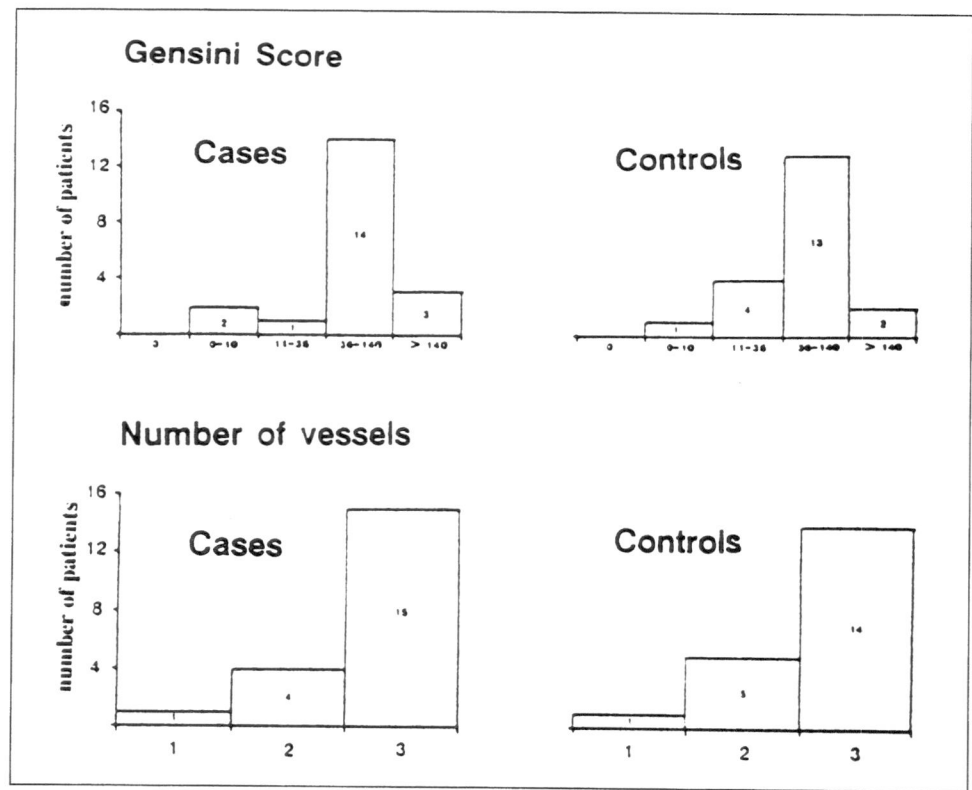

Fig. 1. Extent of coronary lesions in group I (unstable angina and group II (stable angina)

score group I: 98.1, ±54.3, group II: 76.3, ±48.8, p = n.s.). There was no significant difference concerning the risk factors, hypercholesterinemia, smoking, hypertension, diabetes mellitus, and positive family history.

Five patients of group I (UAP) had a new onset angina without preliminary symptoms. The rest reported anginal chest pain of 4 — 96 months duration (mean 35.4, ±29.9), which did not differ significantly from the control group (3—240 months, 240 month? (that's 20 years) Should this be 24 months? mean 44.7, ±53.1, p = n.s.).

Table 1 shows that patients with unstable angina pectoris had not only a change in symptoms, but that their absolute degree of angina pectoris was much more severe than in the control group with stable angina pectoris.

As a special method of assessment of life events we used the "Inventory of life events (ILE)" by Siegrist, published in 1983 [11]. It contains a list of 34 items of different life events and one undefined item for events that are not included in the list. This list includes, e.g., severe physical disease, abortion, death of a member of the family, examinations, several job troubles. These events are to be explored by the investigator. The second part consists of self-rating scales to estimate the subjective stress of every experienced event. Two statements in this part shall determine when the event took place and whether it was a repeated experience or not.

Another nine statements have to be evaluated by the patients as to whether they are correct or not and to what extent they accurately describe the actual situation. These statements describe, for instance, whether there was social support or whether the event interrupted the everyday routine. A score was derived by summing up the respective values of each statement. The sum of the score values for every event ranges from 0—44. Unique experiences, long-lasting stress, and high score values indicate more stress.

Results

We could explore 19 different events: 18 events defined in the ILE and one undefined event were reported by both groups for the intervall of two years before entering the study. In total, there were 41 events reported by both groups, 26 by the

Table 1.

	cases	controls	
angina at			
high physical activity	0/21	8/21	p = 0.0017
minimal physical activity	16/21	8/21	p = 0.014
angina at rest	20/21	7/21	
p = 0.000025 early morning angina	6/21	2/21	n.s.
Frequency of angina pectoris			
< 1× weekly	2/21	13/21	p = 0.00046
1—3× weekly	1/21	2/21	n.s.
4—7× weekly	1/21	3/21	n.s.
> 7× weekly p = 0.00016	17/21	3/21	

patients with UAP (group I), and 15 in group II (controls with stable angina). This difference was significant according to Fischer's exact test ($p = 0.00039$).

If one compares the events with lower subjective stress values of < 20 only, nearly the same amount of events is found in both groups (group I: 15, group II: 13). The significant difference between the two groups is focused on events of a medium- or high-level of subjective stress. The distribution of events with a stress level > 14 is shown in the Table 2.

In the case of our controls (group II), 12 events occurred in the last three months before the beginning of the unstable phase of the illness, and prior to entry in the study. Our definition of cumulation was a minimum stress level of 14.5 which must represent 25% of the whole observation period. UAP patients (group I) showed

Table 2.

Group			Event	
I	Unstable Angina	n = 21	23	p < 0.00005
II	Stable Angina	n = 21	10	

Table 3.

Group			Event	
I	Unstable Angina	n = 21	7	p = 0.022
II	Stable Angina	n = 21	1	

Table 4. Patients with cumulation of life-changing events.

Patient No.		Sum of stress values of events in				% month
		month 1—21		month 22—24		
22—24						
Group I		Event No.		Event No.		
	1	1a	31	25	16	25.4%
		18	20			
	3	1	12	21	18	
		1	12	35	12	42.3%
	4	12	21	26	23	52.3%
	5	—	—	16	16	100.0%
	13	1	8	1	20	71.4%
	15	—	—	20	24	
				1	20	100.0%
	21	16	21	31	19	
		3	23			30.2%
Group II						
	29	13	12	7	23	65,7%

36

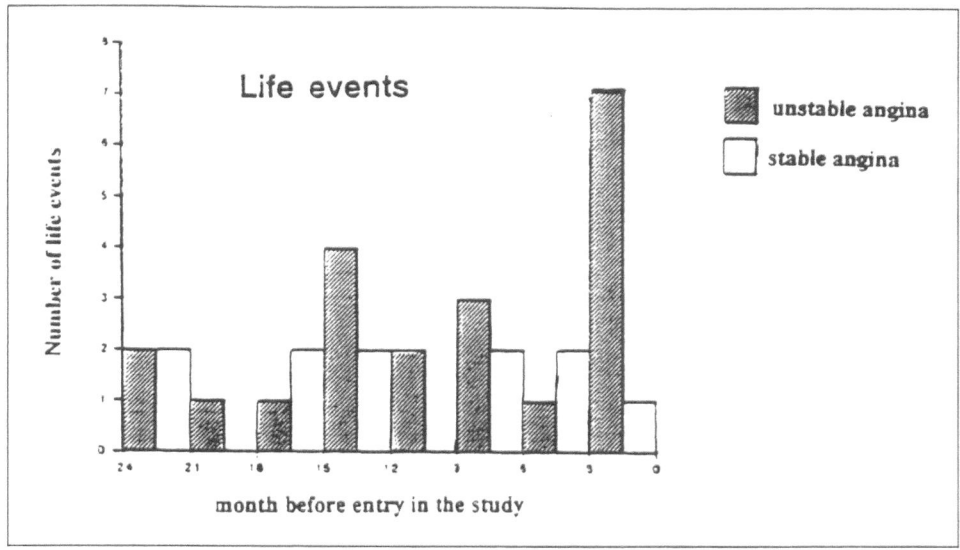

Fig. 2. Distribution of live events of a medium- or high-stress value

significantly more frequent cumulation of events according to the above mentioned conditions than the controls, as shown in the Tables 3 and 4.

The amount of events of a medium- or high-subjective stress level was distributed relatively homogenously over the different three month periods, but in the group of patients with unstable angina pectoris (UAP) it increased abruptly in the last three months before hospitalization. In contrast, the control group had an even distribution of life-events throughout the period in question (Fig. 2).

Discussion

The first instrument to assess life events was developed by Hawkins and Holmes, (1964), the "Schedule of Recent Experience Questionaire" (SRE) which listed common and frequent life events in a standardized form [4]; the incidence of these events was counted. Further investigations lead to more detailed and more elaborated methods of research for life-events. Brown's "Life Event Schedule" was one of the most important innovations. It consists of a great catalog of well defined and detailed events. Especially trained investigators categorize every event the patient reports, based on an inverview with the patient. This instrument also evaluates the individual strain of the events. We used the ILE from Siegrist and Dittmann, published in 1983, which puts the subjective evaluation of the life event by the patient into the center of interest. They supposed that emotional strain grows, the more intensively and more frequently one is forced by life events to assimilate.

The leading results of our study were:

1) patients with unstable angina pectoris (UAP) experienced more frequent life-events thant those with stable angina pectoris;
2) events of higher subjective stress value were much more frequent in the patients with UAP;
3) in contrast to patients with stable angina pectoris, events of a higher stress level cumulated in the last three months before onset of the unstable phase in the patients with UAP.

One possible mechanism that links psycho-social stress and progression of CHD, leading to an unstable phase of the illness may be vasospasm induced by mental stress. Rosansky could show myocardial ischemia, e.g., induced by public speaking in patients with coronary heart disease [9]. This probably is effected by catecholamine secretion and consecutive vasospasm. A transiently constricted, previously sclerosed artery may change its atherosclerotic shape, for example, by plaque rupture; intermittent thrombosis could be a consequence.

There is no way to control the frequency of life events, but prevention of their detrimental effects on patients should be our goal. Severe stressful experiences exhaust the individual's ability to cope. This ability may be strengthened by special training or by better social support to suppress possible unhealthy effects of life-events.

References

1. Davison, Neale (1979) Psychophysiologische Störungen. In: Davison, Neale (eds) Klinische Psychologie. Urban & Schwarzenberg. p 167
2. Gensini G (1979), Cardiac Angiografy, Boston, Mass
3. Jacob A, Spilken A, Norman M (1970) Life stress and respiratory illness. Psychosom Med. 32: 233
4. Joraschky, Köhle (1979) Die Bedeutung von Lebensveränderungen für die Krankheitsmanifestation. In: v. Uexküll (ed) Psychosomatische Medizin. Urban & Schwarzenberg
5. Katschnik H (1980) Methodische Probleme der Life-Event Forschung. Nervenarzt 51: 332
6. Parkes C, Benjamin B, Fitzgerald R (1969) Broken Heart: A statistical study of increased mortality among widowers. Brit Med J 1: 740
7. Rahe R, Lind E (1971) Psychosocial factors and sudden cardiac death: A pilot study J Psychosom Res 25: 19
8. Rahe R, Paasikivi J (1971) Psychosocial factors and myocardial infarction — II. An outpatient study in Sweden. J Psychosom Res 15: 33
9. Rosansky, A, Bairey C, Krantz D, Friedman J (1988) Mental stress and the induction of silent Myocardial ischemia in patients with coronary artery disease. N Engl J Med 16: 1005
10. Siegrist J (1980) Die Bedeutung von Lebensereignissen für die Entstehung körperlicher und psychosomatischer Erkrankungen. Nervenarzt 51: 313
11. Siegrist J, Dittmann K (1983) Beschreibung des ILE. In: Allmendinger, Schmidt, Wegener (eds) ZUMA-Handbuch sozialwissenschaftlicher Skalen. Mannheim p 28
12. Theorell T, Rahe R (1971) Psychosocial factors and myocardial infarction — An inpatient study in Sweden. J Psychosom Res 15: 25
13. Theorell T, Lind E, Fröberg J (1972) A longitudinal study of 21 subjects with coronary heart disease: Life changes, catecholamine excretion and related biochemical reactions. Psychosom Med 34: 505

14. Theorell T (1973) Psychosocial factors and mycocardial infarction — why and how. Adv Cariol 8: 117
15. Wolf S (1969) Psychosocial forces in myocardial infarction and sudden death. Circulation Suppl IV 39: 40

Authors' address:
H. W. Gerbig,
Klinikum Großhadern
Medizinische Klinik I
Marchioninistr. 15
8000 München 70, FRG

Discussion

KRUCOFF:

We can now open this very interesting paper for questions.

GOHLKE:

You made a recommendation to us which I would like to ask you to further elucidate. How should we react? What about psychosocial or psychological counseling for these patients?

GERBIG:

I think that one of the main ways to make events easier for patients is the social support. If the doctor has a good relationship with his patients, he can see him more often after a severe event has occurred and he can be one part of a social support system. It is not possible to reduce the incidence of life events, so one can only help patients to cope with them.

KRUCOFF:

The data you have shown are very intriguing. I think the conclusion to treat patients who face major life events and have known coronary disease with medications, almost in a way to prevent their shift into an unstable pattern, is perhaps one that we should discuss a little more. I think in the United States if you open that door you will have a lot of angioplasty doctors running after death registers, and things might get out of hand in a way that perhaps is not quite the conclusion that you want to come to. Is there, in fact, any hard data to suggest that the sensitivity and specificity of the correlations you have shown, the acceleration of angina or the frequency of life events ant the acceleration of angina, is so sensitive and specific that you would really suggest going ahead and prophylactically treating these people for their coronary disease?

GERBIG:

We have also found patients with stable angina pectoris with severe life events, who lost their jobs, and so on, so you cannot say that everybody reacts in the same way and goes into the unstable phase of the disease. So there are, rather, other reasons why they come into this unstable phase. But, if you know the patient and have personal contact to him and see that he has problems, one has to see whether he is one of the patients who reacts in this way and ask him whether the symptoms of angina pectoris have increased or not. I think a life event cannot be the only cause of an unstable phase of angina pectoris.

MATHES:

There is a universal need for patients to explain the reasons for their infarct or their recent onset of unstable angina. From the desire of the patient to get some reasoning into his disease, we must be very careful about drawing the conclusion that these life events really are the causes or related to the cause of the progression of the disease. What is really needed to make the data more clear is to take a cohort, such as people living in the area of your hospital, and to make a prospective study. This would take away the criticism that has often been uttered. Then your recommendations would be on a much safer ground.

SIEGRIST:

Some years ago we did a study on several hundred patients with premature acute myocardial infarction and a matched control group. We asked their subjective opinion about disease etiology and we found that even if we controlled for the type of disease etiology and if we adjust for neuroticism and other psychological confounders, we still come out with an increased proportion of life events in cases vs controls. I fully agree that we have to do prospective studies, but prospective studies are very expensive and long-lasting, and I think as there is convincing evidence, we should not wait for 10 years to go into intervention. I think the general message is to increase the sensibility of physicians when talking to their patients, to be aware of these problems.

GOHLKE:

Could you tell us again what was the percentage of patients in the unstable group in whom a higher incidence of life events occurred in comparison to the control group?

GERBIG:

I can tell you the percentage of patients who showed a cumulation: that was 30 % vs in cases only 5 % in the controls.

MASERI:

I think that you should be congratulated for having tackled this problem in the way you did, because I think that some of the objections that were raised were answered by the fact that you had these matched controls, and that in the unstable patients you had the control of the previous 24 months showing that there was something happening more closely to the events. I think that in a way you were as careful as one could be with retrospective studies. The problem comes at two levels. At first it is not only a matter of events that happen, it is the way the individual can cope or not cope with the events. Certainly a trauma for one person gives a certain amount of suffering that is not the same for another. Somebody can lose his job and he says, "Well, I lost my job, but that is not the end of the world, I will find another one." Somebody else loses his job and says, "My God, I'm finished, I'm nobody, my life is over, I'm ruined, I want to die." I wonder how this can be taken into consideration.

The second point is the very fact that you are talking about unstable angina. Unstable angina by the definition that we currently accept is something that starts suddenly and unexpectedly. So it would be very difficult to have counseling of patients because unstable angina and often myocardial infarction just come "out of the blue", like an ulcer can come out of the blue. Similarly, somebody with chronic stable angina will not necessarily develop the chronic crescendo type all of a sudden. How do you get to those patients? How do you know whether they are going to develop depression, ulcerative colitis, ulcer, cancer, a cold, unstable angina, or infarction? It becomes very difficult. As a starting point let us see if there is more objective evidence than the clinical impression that I personally have that the phenomena exist. We need a better way to deal with and measure both the stressor and the stress of the individual. Then one can go into prospective studies, because that is obviously the direction to go.

GERBIG:

I perfectly agree with the second part, but I want to answer the first question you asked. You asked whether we also measured the stress level of every individual event. The mere occurence of an event does not say what stress it is. Part of the inventory we used was to measure the subjective stress of the individual. There were criteria, as I mentioned, like social support, or whether it was an event that happened the first time. These criteria go into the stress value.

KRUCOFF:

I think that has been independently confirmed. Alan Rozanski and the Cedars Sinai group actually designed their protocol in the reverse and compelled a patient to stand up in front of an audience and focus on his or her own most embarassing moment or something they found very hard to talk about. They found this stress to be the most profound stimulus of ischemia of all of the stimuli they measured. So I think the point is very real, and I thought the data you showed accounting for the stress level carried that point home.

Sleep disturbances in pre-infarction patients

J. Siegrist

Department of Medical Sociology Medical School, University of Marburg, FRG

Introduction

In two ways, disturbed sleep is likely to indicate a condition of increased pathophysiologic vulnerability in patients with cardiovascular risk factors or clinical manifestation of cardiovascular disease. First, advanced cardiovascular pathophysiology can be seen as a relevant cause of disturbed sleep. It is well known that pain associated with nocturnal unstable angina provokes awakenings, and similar experiences happen in patients with severe peripheral artery occlusion. Poor sleep is often reported in patients with congestive heart failure and may be present in other cardiovascular syndromes. Second, disturbed sleep by itself may promote cardiovascular dysfunction and contribute to the development of breakdown in adaptive responses of the cardiovascular system to internal or external demands. The present contribution focuses on the second approach. After a brief examination of the epidemiologically established link between disturbed sleep and cardiovascular morbidity and mortality two arguments are presented in more detail. The first concentrates on the role of sleep apnea as a risk factor for near-future ischemic heart disease (IHD) whereas the second argument defines distrubed sleep in the framework of chronic social stress which by now is a widely accepted precipitating factor in the development of overt IHD.

Several large scale, longitudinal studies have reported an association between sleep disturbances and subsequent cardiovascular excess morbidity or mortality. A six-year follow-up of a very large sample of adults conducted by the American Cancer Society revealed a relative risk of 2,8 in men sleeping 4 h or less as compared to those sleeping 7—8 h per night. This excess mortality was found for ischemic heart disease, stroke, suicide, and cancer and was established by multiple discriminant analysis after controlling for a large set of possibly confounding variables [13]. The study also found cardiovascular excess mortality of 1.8 in those sleeping more than 10 h. The same trend was evident in the Alameda County Study in which approximately 7000 adults were followed over nine years. The mortality rate for IHD was 1.7 in those sleeping less than 7 h or more than 9 at entry as compared to those with 7—8 h regular sleeping time. There was still a significant excess mortality of poor or long sleepers after controlling for 12 moderating variables [28].

Sleep disturbances, to some extent, were predictive of future cases or myocardial infarction in the Kaiser Permanent Epidemiologic Study [4]. A further study investigated the effect of "tiredness" in different occupations on the incidence of hospitalization during a one year follow-up in Sweden. For women aged 20—54, occupations with a high percentage of members who were markedly tired "during the last two weeks" showed a significantly elevated incidence of hospitalization for myocardial infarction among others [27]. The Finnish Twin Cohort Study included information on sleep habits in about 5400 male twin pairs. It should be mentioned that the study was not prospective but established a significant effect of quality of sleep on the history of pain of possible myocardial infarction by means of multiple logistic regression analysis [17].

Very recently, the same group presented findings from a six-year follow-up study of 10 778 persons aged 35—59 years where poor quality of sleep was associated with life dissatisfaction, stress of daily activities, unemployment, and neuroticism. Age-adjusted risk ratios for bad sleep quality as compared to good quality were calculated for men and women using death certificates and hospital records as criteria. Among other findings, the study could demonstrate a significantly increased risk ratio of for ischemic heart disease (death or hospitalization; [12] 2.04 for men and 2.23 for women.

Taken together, this information shows that poor sleep is associated with a moderately increased risk of future cardiovascular morbidity or mortality. In addition, it shows that somatic as well as psychosocial conditions are involved in the association between sleep disturbances and cardiovascular morbidity [2]. Yet, few, if any, prospective epidemiologic studies have included polysomnographic registration or clinical screening; we are therefore left with considerable uncertainty about the nature of possible links between both phenomena. In the next sections, two approaches towards analyzing those links are outlined.

Sleep apnea in pre-infarction individuals

Sleep apnea is defined as a recurrent nocturnal breathing disorder which causes multiple episodes of temporal cessation of breathing during sleep resulting in a significant decrease of blood oxygen saturation and in a compensating arousal reaction with sudden sympatho-adrenergic stimulation, rapid change from bradycardia to tachycardia, and a rise in pulmonary and systemic arterial blood pressure. Sleep fragmentation in apnoeic patients causes excessive daytime sleepiness — one of the leading subjective symptoms of this disorder — and a general decrease in the level of energy, vigilance, and achievement. A common operational definition of sleep apnea requires the existence of 10 or more apnoeic episodes lasting more than 10 seconds each per hour sleeping time or a total of more than 100 apnoeic episodes during total sleeping time as documented by polysomnographic registration for at leat one night [7].

Multiple strains and arousals recurring over months and years during sleep have potent pathophysiologic consequences, especially so in individuals whose cardiovascular system is already impaired. The following clinical conditions have been investigated in a large number of studies.

1) *Development of systemic hypertension:* At least every third hypertensive patient suffers from sleep apnea [16], and 60—80 % of sleep apnea patients in clinical samples exhibit hypertension [16]. Prevalence of arterial hypertension in a large field study was found to be five times as high in otherwise healthy apnoeic male workers as compared to non-apnoeic workers [15]. It was also shown that sucessful treatment of sleep apnea resulted in blood pressure normalization [6, 18]. Despite this evi-

dence, the pathophysiologic link between sleep apnea activity and persistent high blood pressure is not established so far, and prospective evidence is still scare.

2) *Development of angina pectoris and myocardial infarction:* Hypoxia during apnoeic episodes eventually causes myocardial ischemia resulting in selected cell necrosis. Sudden changes between bradycardia and tachycardia during apnea often trigger cardiac arrhythmias, especially so in a compromised myocardium. Cardiac arrhythmias may contribute to an ischemic myocardium which in turn aggravates the severity of arrhythmias [7; 18, 20].

There is now good evidence from a large prospective study on an association between habitual snoring (as a valid proxy measure of sleep apnea [11, 20]) and the incidence of anginal attacks as well as of fatal or non-fatal acute myocardial infarction. The relative risk of angina pectoris for habitual snoring men was 2.2. and the age-adjusted relative risk of IHD between snorers and non-snorers in this cohort of 4388 men followed over three years was 1.9; if reported history of angina pectoris on myocardial infarction at the beginning of follow-up was controlled for, the relative risk increased to about 2.7 [11]. Interestingly, the trends were identical for non-fatal and fatal IHD and associations persisted after adjusting for a large number of coronary risk factors.

Sleep apnea causing disrupted sleep and stressing the cardiovascular/cardiorespiratory system by recurrent multiple episodes of disordered breathing must be considered an independent risk factor of angina pectoris, of acute myocardial infarction, and of nocturnal sudden cardiac death. This opens the question on the prevalence of sleep apnea in adult populations and the magnitude of an associated cardiovascular excess risk. Few studies so far have documented the prevalence of sleep apnea in adult populations. It is well established that being overweight, male, and consuming alcohol present the main risk factors for nocturnal apnea. In unselected male populations the prevalence of nocturnal apnea, documented by questionnaire and validated in subgroups by polysomnographic registration, varies according to these risk factors, but can be assumed to range from 5 % to 15 %. Two recent epidemiologic studies documented a prevalence of 10 % and 15 %, respectively, in employed, healthy men aged between 20 and 60 years in West Germany [19, 20].

One of these studies was performed in our group. Four-hundred-sixteen middle-aged male blue-collar workers (aged 25 to 55 years, mean 40.8 ± 9.6), free from overt IHD at entry, were followed over three years to establish associations between occupational stress and cardiovascular risk status. During second screening, a representative sample of those workers who reported frequent sleep disturbances during the past four weeks underwent ambulant polysomnographic registration for at least one night. When applying the operational definition of sleep apnea mentioned 15 % of the men were considered to suffer from nocturnal apnea. Table 1 compares mean age, weight, and blood pressure between workers with and without sleep disturbances (A vs B) as well as between the group with increased sleep apnea activity and the group without signs of sleep apnea (B1 vs B2). Interestingly, workers with increased sleep apnea activity did not exhibit significantly increased coronary risk factors as compared to workers without sleep apnea but with sleep disturbances [21].

Can we conclude from these findings that apnea-positive workers are not exposed to excess coronary risk? Considering the small number of subjects studied, only a preliminary answer can be given to this question. However, echocardiography per-

44

Table 1. Characteristics of the study population (354 male blue-collar workers) and its subsamples (mean and standard deviation) [21].

	Age (years)	Overweight (Broca) (kg)	Blood pressure (systolic/ diastolic) (mm Hg)	Mean frequency of apneic episodes (lasting at least 10 s each) (N)	Mean apnea index[a]
A Workers without frequently disrupted sleep (n = 276)	41.8±9.7	113.6±14.1	135.2±1.2 88.1±10.6	—	—
B Workers with frequently disrupted sleep (n = 78) Subgroups with polysomnographic registration:	45.7±8.5	114.9±14.7	135.5±16.1 88.3±10.2		
B1: Workers without increased sleep apnea[b] (n = 12)	49.7±4.6	119.5±12.9	141.6±19.1 89.6±12.3	27.1±19.9	3.5±2.3
B2: Workers with increased sleep apnea[b] (n = 8)	48.8±5.1	121.3±13.3	138.0±12.8 90.8± 7.5	97.6±42.7	13.3±6.2
T-test	4.36 p < 0.001 (A vs B)	ns (A vs B)	ns (A vs B)	5.0 p < 0.0001 (BI vs B2)	7.2 p < 0.001 (BI vs B2)

[a] Number of apneic episodes/h sleeping time
[b] ≥ 50 apneic episodes pernight lasting at least 10 s each.

formed in the apnea-positive blue-collar workers revealed enlarged end-diastolic diameters of the left ventricle (64.0 ± 9.5 mm), enlarged diameters of the septum (10.8 ± 0.5 mm), and greater posterior wall thickness (10.2 ± 1.2 mm) [21]. This finding suggests that hypoxemia and recurrent adrenergic activity associated with apneic episodes may promote left-ventricular hypertrophy in the long run even under conditions of moderate volume load. In this context, it should be remembered that left-ventricular hypertrophy is an important risk factor of cardiac death even after correcting for the level of blood pressure. This has been clearly demonstrated in the Framingham Study by Kannel et al. [8].

In conclusion, sleep apnea has a prevalence of 5—15 % in middle-aged male populations. It facilitates the development of arterial hypertension and of left-ventricular hypertrophy independent of volume load. Nocturnal apnea increases the vulnerability of the myocardium to ischemic attacks and, subsequently, to angina and acute myocardial infarction. Finally, malignant arrhythmias may be triggered resulting in nocturnal sudden cardiac death. Given the impressive prevalence of nocturnal apnea and its pathophysiological consequences, screening for cardiovascular high-risk status should include the application of newly developed ambulant-monitoring techniques or at least of sensitive standardized questionnaires measuring symptoms and complaints of sleep apnea.

Distress-induced sleep disturbances in pre-infarction individuals

The epidemiologic evidence quoted in the introductory section suggested an additional pathway between sleep disturbances and increased near-future coronary events: severe socio-emotional distress. Healthy individuals may well be able to cope with severe socio-emotional distress for a longer period. However, after continuing exposure to social stressors or even after aggravation due to uncontrollable life events, coping abilities may decrease, and a vulnerable psychophysiologic state becomes apparent characterized by prolonged irritation, anger, by feelings of sustained hopelessness, and inability to relax. In this situation, aggravated sleep disturbances are likely to occur. They indicate a state of impaired central neuronal regulation due to severe socio-emotional distress (distress-induced sleep disturbances [24]). This state of impaired central neuronal regulation becomes an important target for further exploration in individuals who are already at cardiovascular risk.

It is known that sleep and cardiovascular function, to some extent, are regulated by common morphological structures such as the brain reticular formation [14]. It is also known that serotonin in the nerve endings of nucleus tractus solitarii is involved in the control of circulation as well as in the control of NREM-sleep [10]. These and other examples indicate that aggravated sleep disturbances may be interpreted as a sign of impaired neuronal regulation within these common centers.

Impaired neuronal regulation may decrease the cardiovascular responsiveness to internal and external stimuli and inhibit lower levels of heart rate during the restoring phases of sleep.

Preliminary ambulant monitoring data collected by the Holter System Oxford 4000 indicate that the regular diurnal pattern observed in healthy persons (clear decrease of mean heart rate during sleep in the condensed time pattern) is leveled off [24]. Heart rate activity continues to be elevated even during the restoring phases of sleep. This elevated cardiac activity during sleep can contribute to myocardial vulnerability in high risk people. Clinical studies in patients with ischemic heart disease have shown that administration of a calcium antagonist which depletes noradrenaline terminals and inhibits excessive sympathetic arousal has beneficial effects on the patterning of heart rate in the day-night cycle [5], i. e., on a decrease of heart rate during sleep [5].

A decrease in the modulation of cardiovascular response to external or internal stimuli has been linked to the down-regulation of hormonal receptors as a consequence of chronic stress [1, 3, 22]. If this holds true decreased cardiovascular responsiveness should be expected as well during daytime challenge in those individuals who suffer from severe chronic social stress. We tested this hypothesis in the framework of our prospective study. During the third screening of the blue-collar population a standardized psychomental stress test — a modified version of the Stroop colour-word-interference test — was performed at the end of a work day. Blood pressure and heart rate reactions were measured (see [9, 22]). Analysis of

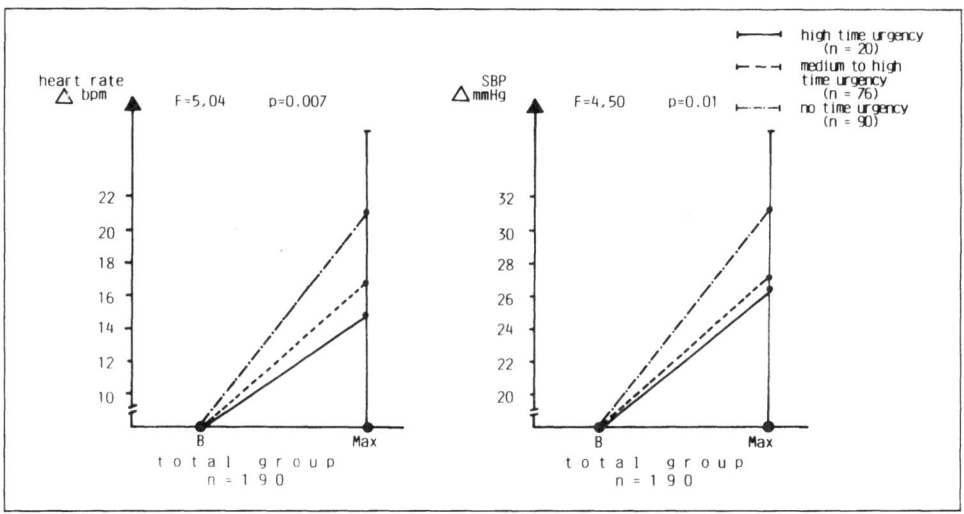

Fig. 1. Difference in heart rate (HR) reaction and in systolic blood pressure (SBP) between baseline (B) and maximal stress (max) according to degree of chronic occupational stress (time urgency), adjusted for age and smoking (STROOP colour word conflict task)

variance adjusting for the effects of age, of hypertensive status, and of smoking revealed significant main effects of indicators of chronic occupational stress on cardiovascular responsiveness (in Fig. 1, as an example, chronic occupational stress is measured by "high time urgency at work").

A summary of findings consistent with this pattern is forthcoming [9]. It supports the notion of impaired neuronal regulation of cardiovascular responsiveness during sleep and wakefulness in individuals who suffer from severe chronic social stress. Whereas the clinical significance of these findings is not clear so far, first results from the prospective study, based on small numbers, show that subjects who during their last interview reported severe sleep-disturbances were at a higher risk of developing their first fatal or non-fatal myocardial infarction within the two subsequent years as compared to those with normal sleep. The relative risk was 3.8 in those reporting frequent early wakenings in the morning without falling asleep again and 2.6 in those reporting frequent difficulties staying asleep during the night. As these findings are based on small numbers it will be important to extend such studies to larger sample groups and longer observation periods.

Elsewhere, we have shown that conditions which provoke severe socio-emotional distress in working men such as increase of workload, high-time urgency, tensions with co-workers, inability to promote one's career, and low occupational status are all correlated with the frequency of reported sleep disturbances [23]. The same holds true for a critical pattern of coping with the demands at work ("need for control", especially its latent factor, "immersion"). This critical pattern of coping termed "immersion" was found to be significantly higher in patients with myocardial infarction as compared to healthy men, and was also significantly increased in men waiting for coronary bypass surgery [26].

Table 2: Analysis of variance: mean score of "immersion" in male workers with severe sleep disturbances (SSD) vs undisturbed sleep, correcting for age.

	Score "immersion" mean sd	F	2-tailed p	T separate estimate	2-tailed p
Workers with SSD (n = 57)	4.86 ± 2.22				
Workers without SSD (n = 211)	3.15 ± 1.96	1.29	0.208	− 5.26	0.0001

Table 2 shows that a group of workers defined by severe sleep disturbances exhibits a significantly higher mean score on the scale measuring "immersion" compared to men without sleep disturbances. The statistical effect persists after correcting for the influence of age on sleep disturbances.

The findings reported indicate that distress-induced sleep disturbances deserve more attention in future studies on an association between disrupted sleep and near-future ischemic events. Both approaches analyzed in this paper may help to improve identification of cardiovascular high-risk individuals and thus contribute to cardiovascular prevention.

References

1. Anisman H, Kokkinidis L, Sklar LS (1984) Neurochemical consequences of stress. In: Burchfield SK (ed) Stress, psychological and physiological interactions. Hemisphere Publ, Washington, pp 67—97
2. Appels A, de Vos J, van Diest R, Höppener P, Mulder P, de Groen J (1987) Are sleep complaints predictive of future myocardial infarction? Act Nerv (Suppl) 29: 147—151
3. Axelrod J, Reisine TD (1984) Stress hormones: Their interaction and regulation. Science 242: 452—459
4. Friedman GD, Ury HK, Klatsky AL (1974) A psychological questionnaire predictive of myocardial infarction: results from the Kaiser permanente epidemiologic study of myocardial infarction. Psychosom Med 36: 327—343
5. Guerchicoff S, Drager S, Kunik M, Vazquez A (1988) Antiarrhythmic effect of prenylamine. In: Manning AS, Szendey CL (eds) Prenylamine: a novel approach to myocardial protection. Raven Press, New York, pp 109—114
6. Guilleminault C, Cummisky J, Dement WC (1980) Sleep apnea syndromes: recent advances. Adv Intern Med 26: 347—372
7. Guilleminault, C., Dement WC (eds) (1978) Sleep apnea syndromes. AR LISS, New York, pp 177—196
8. Kannel WS, Sorlie P (1981) Left ventricular hypertrophy in hypertension: prognostic and pathogenetic implication (the Framingham study). In: Strauer BE (ed) The heart in hypertension. Springer Berlin Heidelberg New York pp 223—241
9. Klein D (1988) Kardiovaskuläre Belastungsreaktionen bei Industriearbeitern. Doctoral Dissertation University of Marburg
10. Koella WP (1984) The organization and regulation of sleep. Experientia 40: 309—338

11. Koskenvuo M, Kaprio J, Telakivi T, Partinen M, Heikkilä K, Sarna S (1987) Snoring as a risk factor for ischemic heart disease and stroke in men. In: Peter J, Podszus T, von Wichert P (eds) Sleep related disorders and internal diseases. Springer Berlin Heidelberg New York pp 211—218

12. Koskenvuo M, Kaprio J, Partinen M, Langinvainio H, Sarna S, Rita H, Heikkilä K (1988) Poor sleep quality, emotional stress and morbidity (to be published)

13. Kripke DF, Simons RN, Garfinkel L, Hammond EC (1979) Short and long sleep and sleeping pills. Is increased morbidity associated? Arch Gen psychiatry 36: 103—116

14. Langhorst P, Schulz G, Lambertz M, Krienke B (1980) Funktionelle Organisation eines gemeinsamen Hirnstammsystems für Kreislauf, Atmung und allgemeine Aktivitätsmessung. In: Schiffer R (ed) Zentralvegetative Regulationen und Syndrome. Springer, Berlin Heidelberg New York, pp 39—55

15. Lavie P (1983) Sleep apnea in industrial workers. In: Guilleminault C, Lugaresi E (eds) Sleep-wake disorders: natural history, epidemiology and longterm evolution. Raven, New York pp 127—135

16. Lavie P (1987) Rediscovering sleepy patients: the sleep apnea syndrome. In: Peter J, Podszus T, von Wichert P (eds) Sleep related disorders and internal diseases. Springer Berlin Heidelberg New York pp 227—240

17. Partinen M, Putkonen PTS, Kaprio J, Koskenvuo M, Hilakivi I (1982) Sleep disorders in relation to coronary heart disease. Acta Med Scand (Suppl) 660: 69—83

18. Peter JH (1987) Die Erfassung der Schlafapnoe in der Inneren Medizin. Thieme, Stuttgart

19. Peter JH, Hess U, Himmelmann H, Köhler U, Mayer J, Podszus T, Siegrist J, Sohn E (1987) Sleep apnea activity and general morbidity in a field study. In: Peter JH, Podszus T, von Wichert P (eds) Sleep related disorders and internal diseases. Springer, Berlin Heidelberg New York, pp 248—253

20. Peter J, Podszus T, von Wichert P (eds) (1987) Sleep related disorders and internal diseases. Springer, Berlin Heidelberg New York

21. Peter JH, Siegrist J, Podszus T, Mayer J, Selzer K, von Wichert P (1985) Prevalence of sleep apnea in healthy industrial workers. Klin Wochenschr. 63: 807—811

22. Sapolski RM, Krey LC, McEwen SB (1984) Stress down-regulates corticosteron receptors in a site-specific manner in the brain. Endocrinology 114: 287—298

23. Siegrist J (1987) Impaired quality of life as a risk factor in cardiovascular disease. J Chron Dis 40: 571—578

24. Siegrist J (1987) Sleep disturbances and cardiovascular risk. In: Peter J, Podszus T, von Wichert P (eds) Sleep related disorders and internal diseases. Springer, Berlin Heidelberg New York, pp 173—182

25. Siegrist J, Klein D, Matschinger H (1988) Occupational distress, coronary risk factors and cardiovascular responsiveness. In: Weiner H, Hendrie D, Florin I, Hellhammer D (eds) New fontiers in stress research. Huber, Bern Toronto (forthcoming)

26. Siegrist J, Matschinger H (1988) Distress-Karriere und koronares Risiko. Jahrbuch für Medizinische Psychologie, Springer, Berlin Heidelberg New York 1: 87—99

27. Theorell T, Akerstedt T, Alfredsson L, Spetz CL (1988) Tired occupations and hospitalization (to be published)

28. Wingard DL, Berkman LF (1983) Mortality risk associated with sleeping pattern among adults. Sleep 6: 102—107

Author's address:
Prof. Dr. J. Siegrist
Department of Medical Sociology
Medical School, University of Marburg,
Bunsenstraße 2
D-3550 Marburg, FRG

Discussion

MASERI:

This is a very interesting angle from which to look at the problem. I would just like to bring out the fact that you have basically two kinds of sleep apnea: one, where there is no stimulation of the motoneurons of the inspiratory muscles. The other is the one where you do have the stimulation of the respiratory muscles, there are efforts to breathe, and yet the glottis is closed, and this is typical of people that have one kind of pickwickian syndrome, which is probably related to two factors: one, fat accumulation around the glottis, and two, weakness of the pharyngeal muscles — so that probably is a different thing from the one where there are stimuli that just suppress the rhythmicity of the respiratory center. There the problem comes that the same stimuli that may inhibit the respiratory center may also, perhaps on some other occasions or in some other way, have have an excitatory effect on the cardiovascular center, which is not far away, anatomically, from the respiratory center. It is a very intriguing angle from which you propose that we should look at this problem.

SIEGRIST:

I fully agree that further studies have to differentiate the types of apnea. However, if we go into the prevalence rates of the different types, obstructive, non-obstructive, and so on, we find that the pickwickian type has a rather low prevalence. A much higher prevalence of sleep apnea is found in apparently healty middle-aged men, of course a little bit obese, a little bit hypertensive, perhaps prone to alcohol consumption, but otherwise healthy. They are not the classic pickwician type. I think that what I showed was mainly confined to this type, and should differentiate more into subclusters. But as you know, it is also difficult in terms of assessing and monitoring. We did some monitoring in the blue-collar study with polysomnographic ambulant monitoring. Very unexpectedly, we found that among those who indicated on our questionnaires recurrent severe sleep disturbances, 15% showed severe sleep apnea, and were not aware of that. So the prevalence of this problem may be a critical point.

FOX:

We were interested in this problem: we were looking at patients with severe angina and we studied them in a sleep laboratory. We had one patient who developed 40-s periods of apnea; this was associated with the development of a tachydardia, a fall in PO2, and the development of myocardial ischemia on the ECG with marked ST segment depression, and then the patient awakened with chest pain. We also found that the changes in the phase of sleep, from phase 4 to phase 3 to phase 2, were associated as they lightened their phase of sleep with a tachycardia and the subsequent development of ischemia. I wonder if people who have life events, are not changing their phases of sleep much more than people who do not, and therefore, are developing periods of tachycardia more frequently through the night than otherwise. I would be interested in your comments on that.

SIEGRIEST:

The first comment is that due to the time urgency of this presentation I was not concentrating on the types of arrhythmias which are found in sleep-apneic patients. There is one very critical shift, and that is the shift from bradycardia to tachycardia associated with the arousal reaction. In a compromised myocardium it might well be that exactly at this phase the malignant arrythmias occur, and nocturnal sudden death might be one of the consequences — of course only in individuals with advanced pathology. Secondly, I think we are not yet in a position to answer this question, to say this is a subgroup who experienced severe life events, and not only severe in terms of common-sense judgment, but in terms of this assessment technique which takes into account the subjective evaluation in terms of stress dimensions. We are planning a further study in which we would like to include hormonal assessment and ambulatery ECG monitoring in those sociologically and psychologically high-risk groups.

The association between vital exhaustion, unstable angina, and future myocardial infarction

A. Appels and C. F. Mendes De Leon

Dept. Medical Psychology, Rijksuniversiteit Limburg, The Netherlands

Introduction

The identification of an impending heart attack remains one of the major challenges of clinical and preventive cardiology. Several cardiologists, therefore, studied the symptoms and complaints most often experienced by coronary victims shortly before acute myocardial infarction (MI) or sudden cardiac death. It was found that the most commonly reported premonitory symptoms include chest pain, dyspnea, excess fatigue, lack of energy, or a feeling of general malaise. The prevalence estimates of excess fatigue prior to acute MI or cardiac death differ from study to study, and vary between 30% and 50%. This was equal to or larger than the prevalence of other prodromal symptoms [7, 8, 10, 11]. Most cardiologists would probably avoid interpretation of these feelings of "excess fatigue" or "lack of energy," or are inclined to interpret these feelings as being related to angina pectoris, medication, or aging.

According to our clinical experience, feelings of excessive tiredness can only be partially attributed to a deteriorated somatic condition or medication. Angina pectoris or some anti-hypertensive drugs may cause fatigue, but these factors cannot fully account for the high prevalence of excessive tiredness among coronary-prone individuals. Therefore, we made a detailed analysis of these feelings and tested the hypothesis that they constitute an independent risk factor of coronary heart disease.

In this report we will first briefly describe the nature of the psychological precursors of acute myocardial infarction. Next, we will present some data of a prospective study of 3 877 males and of a case-control study of patients hospitalized because of unstable angina pectoris. We will end with a discussion of the physiological mechanisms which possibly explain the relationship between exhaustion and ischemic heart disease endpoints.

Vital exhaustion

A large number of interviews were conducted with coronary patients in order to gain more insight into the exact nature of the feelings of tiredness preceding MI. The interviews revealed that the excess fatigue or lack of energy preceding MI reflected a state of mental and physical exhaustion. Patients reporting that they had experienced such feelings most often complained of a loss of vitality, listlessness, loss of libido, and increased irritability. Patients often express these feelings in methaphors, such as: "The well is drying out", or "My body is like a battery that is losing its power". They frequently attribute these feelings to a longstanding problem that they have been unable to solve, or to a real or a symbolic loss. It should be noted that such feelings describe a state quite similar to minor depression or demoralization. Coronary patients usually do not report a decrease in selfesteem or the presence of guilt feelings which makes this state distinct from clinical depression. This led us to label these feelings as a state of "vital exhaustion" [1].

The self-descriptions of the coronary patients were used to construct a scale, labeled the Maastricht Questionnaire (MQ). Typical items of the MQ include: "Do you believe that you have come to a dead end?"; "Do you feel like you want to give up trying?"; "Do you feel dejected?"; "Do you feel that your body is like a battery that is losing its power?"; "Do you often feel tired?". The total scale (form A of the MQ) consisted of 37 items. This scale was used to test the hypothesis that vital exhaustion increases the risk for future MI [3].

Vital Exhaustion as a Risk Factor for Coronary Heart Disease

A prospective study was conducted among civil servants of the city of Rotterdam, the Rotterdam Civil Servant Study (RCSS). The cohort of this study was composed of 3 877 male subjects, aged 39—65 years old. Medical examination at screening included measurement of blood pressure, cholesterol, glucose tolerance, relative weight, smoking habits, and assessment of the prevalence of angina pectoris (AP) using the Rose Questionnaire. A resting electrocardiogram completed the cardiovascular screening [3].

Two-hundred-and-seventy subjects (5%) were identified at screening as suffering from AP, of whom 73% scored in the upper tertile of the MQ-scores. Another 47 subjects were identified with unstable AP, of whom 87% scored in the upper tertile of the MQ-scores. Unstable AP was defined by the presence of anginal complaints of recent onset or of increasing frequency and/or severity. Fifty-five subjects had a history of MI.

Subjects were grouped into the lower two tertiles (the "vital" group) or the upper tertile of the MQ (the "exhausted" group) in order to compute the association between the MQ and heart disease at screening. Table 1 shows that the age-adjusted relative risks were 3.05 for stable AP and 17.21 for unstable AP. These relative risks

Table 1. Age-adjusted association between vital exhaustion and past or present heart disease at screening in the Rotterdam Civil Servants Study.

	Odds Ratio	95% CI	X^2 mh
Angina pectoris	3.05	2.26— 4.11	53.60*
Unstable angina	17.21	8.05—36.83	53.82*
Prior myocardial infarction	1.22	0.72— 2.06	0.55

* $p < 0.001$

Table 2. Age-adjusted association between vital exhaustion and future manifestations of coronary heart disease in the Rotterdam Civil Servants Study.

	Relative Risk	95% CI	X^2 mh
Angina pectoris	1.86	1.10—3.15	5.40*
Non-fatal myocardial infarction	2.28	1.22—4.25	6.68**
Fatal myocardial infarction	1.39	0.59—3.25	0.56

* p < 0.05; ** p < 0.01

were highly significant (p < 0.01), and remained unchanged after adjustment for either cholesterol, blood pressure, or smoking. No significant association was found between MQ-scores and history of MI.

The particularly strong association between vital exhaustion and unstable angina is noteworthy, although the cross-sectional nature of the data obviously precludes a causal interpretation of this finding. It indicates that the vast majority of subjects sampled from an open population and identified with unstable AP on the basis of an interview-method feel exhausted.

During follow-up, 38 non-fatal MIs and 21 fatal MIs were documented among the subjects free of CHD at screening. New angina, defined as documented angina, bypass surgery, or possible MI occurred among 54 participants. As shown in Table 2, scores in the upper tertile of the MQ were significantly associated with increased risk for future AP (RR = 1.86) and future non-fatal MI (RR = 2.28). No significant relationship was observed between MQ-scores and future fatal MI. The relative risks remained largely unchanged after adjustment for cholesterol, blood pessure, and smoking. Logistic regressions, with the MQ introduced as a continuous variable into the equation and AP or MI as dependent variable, basically confirmed these results. The equations for both AP and MI as disease end-points produced logistic regression coefficients significant at the p = 0.01 level, after controlling for age, cholesterol, blood pressure, and smoking [3].

These results indicate that vital exhaustion increases the risk for AP and non-fatal MI, independent of the classic risk factors. Analysis of the observed associations against length of the time interval showed a sharp decrease in the relative risk for a hard coronary event (documented MI or cardiac death) occurring in the first, second, third, and fourth year of follow-up. The age-adjusted relative risks associated with a score above the median of the MQ for the first to the fourth year of follow-up are 10.05, 2.23, 3.04, and 0.68, respectively. These figures are rather inaccurate due to the small number of events and are the reason why the median-split was used in these analyses. They do suggest, however, that vital exhaustion is probably a short-term risk factor [3]. As mentioned above, new cases of AP during follow-up were combined into one group with new cases of possible MI and subjects that underwent bypass surgery. This new definition of AP was used in order to obtain a sufficient amount of cases to analyze through multivariate statistics. This is evidently a rather crude definition of AP. A case-control study by Mendes de Leon provided the opportunity to use a more accurate definition of unstable AP.

Vital exhaustion and unstable angina pectoris

A case-control study was conducted at a state-referral hospital in Texas, USA, in order to cross-validate the Dutch findings with respect to vital exhaustion and ischaemic heart disease [13]. As part of this study, information was collected from 22 patients with unstable angina pectoris (cases) and 44 hospital controls. Cases were defined on the basis of diagnosis at discharge from the hospital. This group was composed of 14 patients diagnosed as having an ICD-9 code of 411.1 (intermediate coronary syndrome) and eight patients with an ICD-9 code of 413.9 (non-Prinz Metal angina pectoris). All patients had been admitted to the hospital for an episode of acute chest pain or episodes of chest pain accelerating in frequency and/or severity, suggestive of coronary ischaemia. Control subjects included a variety of other patients, of whom most were admitted for orthopedic surgery, in particular fracture patients and patients with arthritic conditions. All subjects completed a questionnaire while still in the hospital.

The questionnaire contained a briefer version of the MQ (21 items) and four separate items on sleep dysfunction: "trouble falling asleep"; "waking up two or more times per night"; "trouble staying asleep, including waking up far too early", and "waking up after your usual amount of sleep feeling tired and worn out" [9]. The MQ items referred to the three months prior to hospital admission, whereas the sleep dysfunction items referred to the past month before admission. A total sleep dysfunction score was computed by adding up the scores of the four items.

In terms of background variables, the unstable AP case group and control group were very similar in age (52.6 and 53.1 years old, respectively) and education (10.4 and 10.7 years of completed formal schooling). However, significantly more controls (30%) were not married in comparison with the cases (5%; X-square = 5.49; $p < 0.05$). Univariate analyses (t-test) indicate that unstable AP patients have, on the average, higher MQ-scores than hospitalized control patients (18.9 vs 15.3), but this difference failed to reach statistical significance. However, the unstable AP patients had significantly higher scores on the sleep dysfunction scale than the controls (10.0 vs 6.3; $p < 0.05$). Next, all subjects were categorized in tertiles of MQ scores and sleep dysfunction scores, based on the distribution of those scores in the combined groups. Two logistic regressions were performed with case-status as dependent variable, while the categorized MQ variable and the sleep dysfunction variable were entered separately as dependent variable, in addition to a number of control variables. Control variables included age, education, marital status, and smoking status.

Table 3. Association between vital exhaustion and sleep dysfunction and unstable angina pectoris, as derived from multiple logistic regression, controlling for age, education, marital status, and smoking.

	Odds Ratio*	95% CI	sign.
Exhausted vs Vital**	2.36	0.95—5.88	$p < 0.07$
Most vs Least Sleeping Problems**	2.16	0.87—5.37	$p < 0.10$

* The odds of being associated with.

The results for the MQ scale and the sleep dysfunction scale are presented in Table 3. They show that the upper tertile of the MQ is associated with an almost significant logistic regression coefficient with respect to case-status. It indicates that subjects scoring in the upper tertile of the MQ have a more than two fold increased risk of developing unstable AP compared with subjects scoring in the lowest tertile (Odds Ratio = 2.36; p < 0.07). There was also an increased risk for unstable angina associated with the upper tertile of the sleep dysfunction in comparison with the lowest tertile, although this association also just failed to reach statistical significance (Odds Ratio = 2.16; p < 0.10). There was no elevated risk for unstable AP associated with the middle tertile of either the MQ or the sleep dysfunction scale in comparison to the lowest tertile. In sum, the results of this case-control study show that feelings of vital exhaustion and sleep dysfunction may be related to unstable patterns of angina. It is perhaps due to the lack of power, considering the fairly small sample size, that some of these associations just failed to reach statistical significance.

Inspection of the separate sleep complaints revealed that the overall association between sleep dysfunction and unstable AP was mainly due to one sleep complaint, i.e., "How often in the past month did you wake up after your usual amount of sleep feeling tired and worn out?". This finding corresponds with the results of the RCSS. Further item-analysis of form A of the MQ showed that particularly the item "Do you ever wake up with a feeling of exhaustion and fatigue?" was predictive of future MI. The predictive power of this item persisted after controlling for items asking for trouble falling asleep and trouble staying asleep. Although the data are rather limited, they suggest that pre-infarction patients may experience more sleep disturbances than a control population. Especially the complaint "waking up exhausted" may have prognostic relevance [2].

Discussion

The main findings of the RCSS support the hypothesis that vital exhaustion is a short-term risk factor for MI. They also indicate that the relationship between vital exhaustion and future MI is not the result of previous manifestations of heart disease and is independent of the other risk factors of CHD, including age, cholesterol, blood pressure, and smoking. These results correspond with findings by Crisp and colleagues, who observed in a prospective study that a state of sadness, coupled with a loss of libido and exhaustion characterized those destined for myocardial infarction [4]. A case-control study by Falger provided further evidence for the validity of the association between vital exhaustion as measured by the MQ and MI [6].

The relationship between vital exhaustion and unstable angina at screening as observed in the RCSS and in the case-control study of Mendes de Leon suggests that similar symptoms, perhaps in combination with sleep disturbances, are predisposing conditions for unstable AP. It should be noted, however, that it still cannot be ruled out that excess tiredness is caused by subclinical levels of cardiac or more general decompensation, and thus explains the association between vital exhaustion and MI. Therefore, any suggestion that exhaustion may be considered as a cause of heart disease should be avoided. A study is currently in progress to examine whether feelings of vital exhaustion can be attributed to extent of coronary atherosclerosis. Alternatively, or additionally, periods of vital exhaustion may be associated with particular physiologic mechanisms which in turn contribute to the sudden onset or progression of ischaemic events. When questioning which mechanisms may explain the observed association, we enter an almost virgin territory. Two studies have started to explore such mechanisms.

In one study, the relationship was examined between vital exhaustion and a number of physiological indices including cardiovascular reactivity and hormonal reactions during a high stress situation [5]. A real life stressor, the defense of a dissertation by Ph.D. candidates, was selected as the high stress condition. Public defence of a Ph.D. thesis in the Netherlands is typically associated with considerable amounts of tension and nervousness, in addition to a very busy schedule. Subjects were tested on the morning of their defense, and measurements included heart rate, blood pressure, noradrenaline, and serum cholesterol. At the same time, they completed a questionnaire with the MQ in addition to a number of other scales. Thirty-three subjects, all male, participated, with a mean age of 35.7 years (S.D. = 7.5). They were retested several weeks later, which served as the control day.

Heart rate, systolic and diastolic blood pressure, adrenaline, and noradrenaline proved to be significantly higher on the day of the defense in comparison with the control day. Although the mean cholesterol level was also higher on the day of defense, this difference was not significant. MQ scores showed a positive association with serum cholesterol levels on the control day (r = 0.37), and with serum cholesterol (r = 0.60) and noradrenaline (r = 0.32) on the high stress day. Moreover, MQ scores were significantly associated with an increase in cholesterol and adrenaline during the high stress condition, with the control day measurements serving as baseline levels. Further analyses with factor analysis revealed that measures of cholesterol and cholesterol change, as well as noradrenaline and noradrenaline change loaded on the same dimension as the MQ scores. Other physiological changes were found to be associated with a factor measuring type-A behavior. These findings suggest, albeit very tentatively, that vital exhaustion exerts its influence on the cardiovascular system through noradrenaline induced free fatty acids mobilization.

A second study explored the relationship between vital exhaustion and catecholamines and platelet aggregation [12]. In that study, 24 male volunteers, on the average 40 years old, were tested during one control session (for baseline measures) and two experimental sessions of high stress (auditory vigilance tasks). According to self-reports, only one of the experimental sessions was experienced as highly stressful. The rank order correlation between MQ-scores and noradrenaline levels (in venous blood) was highly significant (r = 0.51; p < 0.01), but only during the highly stressful condition. The correlation between MQ-scores and noradrenaline was positive but non-significant during the control session (r = 0.24; n.s.). In addition, the association between MQ-scores and change in the number of platelets that had formed reversible aggregates increased with increasing levels of experienced stress during the three sessions (from control session to the low stress-level experimental session to the high stress-level experimental session). Reversely, the association between MQ-scores and changes in freely circulating platelets decreased with increasing levels of experimental stress.

56

These very first results of two explorations about neurohormonal correlates of vital exhaustion make us belief that stressful conditions may enhance the excretion of noradrenaline among vitally exhausted subjects. Increased noradrenaline may both influence the mobilization of cholesterol and the thrombogenic properties of the blood. As mentioned earlier, this domain of research still is an almost virgin territory. The Maastricht Questionnaire may be a useful research instrument to further explore this field.

References

1. Appels A, Höppener P, Mulder P (1987) A questionnaire to assess premonitory symptoms of myocardial infarction. International Journal of Cardiology 17: 15—24
2. Appels A, de Vos Y, van Diest R, Höppener P, Mulder P (1987) Are sleep complaints predictive of future myocardial infarction? Activitas Nervosa Superior 29: 147—151
3. Appels A, Mulder P (1988) Excess fatigue as a precursor of myocardial infarction. European Heart Journal. 9, 750—764
4. Crisp AH, Queenan M, D'Souza M (1984) Myocardial infarction and the emotional climate. Lancet March 17: 616—619
5. van Doornen L (1988) Physiological Stress Reactivity. Its Relationship to Behavioral Style, Mood, Sex, and Aerobic Fitness. Ph. D. Thesis, Free University of Amsterdam, the Netherlands.
6. Falger PRJ, Appels A, Bekkers J (1986) Biographische Analyse und Herzinfarkt, eine Untersuchung an Herzinfarktpatienten und zwei Referenzgruppen. Zeitschrift für Gerontologie 19: 276—285
7. Feinleib M, Simon A, Gillum R, Marjolis J (1975) Prodromal symptoms and signs of sudden death. Circulation Suppl. 51 and 52: 155—159
8. Fraser GE (1978) Sudden death in Auckland. Australian New Zealand Journal of Medicine 8: 490—499
9. Jenkins CD, Stanton BA, Niemcryk SJ, Rose RM (1988) A scale for the estimation of sleep problems in clinical research. Journal of Clinical Epidemiology 41: 313—321
10. Klæboe G, Otterstad JE, Winsnes T, Espeland N (1987) Predictive value of prodromal symptoms in myocardial infarction. Acta Medica Scandinavia 222: 27—30
11. Kuller LH (1978) Prodromata of sudden death and myocardial infarction. Advances in Cardiology 25: 61—72
12. Lulofs R, Stress Reactions in Subjects at Elevated Psychological Risk for Myocardial Infarction. Ph.D. Thesis in preparation, University of Limburg, the Netherlands
13. Mendes de Leon CF (1988) Behavioral and Emotional Precursors of Acute Heart Disease. Ph.D. Thesis, University of Texas Medical Branch, Galveston, TX.

Authors' address:
Prof. Dr. A. Appels
Dept. Medical Psychology,
Rijksuniversiteit Limburg,
P.O.Box 616,
6200 MD Maastricht,
The Netherlands

Discussion

KRUCOFF:

I would like to provoke, if I could, your sense of vital exhaustion and its role as a primary cause of cardiac events vs it as a secondary reflection. Unless there was a correlation with some objective marker beyond just angina as to the activity of ischemic heart disease it would be very hard to feel confident that vital exhaustion was a cause vs a result.

APPELS:

Well, I fully agree, that is why I said any suggestion of vital exhaustion as a cause of the disease should be avoided. Angiography results correlated with scores for vital exhaustion do not show a very strong correlation. Now we are testing just that idea by looking after those who were treated by dilatation. We want to see whether vital exhaustion just after PTCA predicts restenosis.

GOHLKE:

My question is in the same direction as far as, is it a predictor or is it just a manifestation of an otherwise so far clinically inapparent status of the disease? Perhaps it might be helpful if you break down your time interval a little bit further as far as the one-year interval is concerned. If might perhaps become clearer if you break this interval of a year in to quarterly intervals.

APPELS:

I agree that it could be just a reflection of underlying disease, but that is open. I do not believe that a further breakdown of our follow-up period into smaller periods could help us very much, because the number of cases becomes so small and statistical problems arise.

MASERI:

Well, I think I will be on your side, because I am impressed by whatever gives a risk ratio of 10 to one over the first year and the prevalence of this is important. I used to believe that you get myocardial infarction or unstable angina because you had a very gentle graduate progression of coronary disease that culminates in the event. We see too many patients in whom after thrombolysis the lesion that was occluded by the thrombus is a minor one, less than 50%, and the other coronaries are okay. We see at the other extreme patients with chronic stable angina and severe three-vessel disease who after two, three, four years, are still the same. So the two things as not necessarily go hand in hand, and I would hesitate to think that a chronic pre-clinic progression of the disease manifests itself with cardiac symptoms of sub-clinical ischemia before having myocardial infarction. I am more inclined to believe that the event of coronary occlusion is probably related to a combination of many different factors, including bad luck.

Plasminogen activator inhibitor-1 and transient myocardial ischemia

K. Huber[1], I. Lang[1], M. Joerg[2], P. Probst[1], and B. R. Binder[2]

Departments of Cardiology (head: Prof. F. Kaindl) [1] and Clinical Experimental Physiology (head: Prof. B. R. Binder) [2], University of Vienna, Austria

Introduction

Coronary-angiographic studies and autoptic findings [1—10] have demonstrated a major role of coronary thrombus formation in the pathomechanisms leading to acute coronary syndromes like unstable angina and acute myocardial infarction. Furthermore, it has been shown that 30—70% of patients with coronary artery disease (CAD) exhibit elevated levels of the fast-acting inhibitor of tissue plasminogen activator (PAI-1) [11—16]. Therefore, it has been discussed whether these findings might explain an increased thrombotic risk by impairment of the total fibrinolytic potential or whether elevations of PAI-1 levels are age-related [17, 18] or a reactive phenomenon due to recurrent chest pain and other stress factors [19, 20]. Indeed, it has been shown that PAI-1 elevation can be caused by a wide spectrum of diseases which are not related to thromboembolic events [20, 21].

It was the aim of this study to correlate elevations of PAI-1 activities in plasma with the existence of coronary-sclerotic lesions and to investigate whether PAI-1 increase is more likely the cause of or a reaction to transient myocardial ischemia. Therefore, in a preliminary study we compared plasma PAI-1 concentrations in age-matched patients with chronic chest-pain syndrome who suffered either from angiographically proven coronary sclerosis or from vasospastic angina without angiographic evidence of coronary sclerosis. Secondly, patients with unstable angina with or without development of acute myocardial infarction were investigated to prove a possible relationship between time of onset of myocardial ischemia and circadian variations of plasma PAI-1 concentrations. A further study was undertaken to determine whether alterations of PAI-1 plasma levels correlate with onset of renewed chest pain based on coronary restenosis in patients after successful percutaneous transmural coronary angioplasty (PTCA).

Methods

PAI-1 assay

PAI-1 determinations have been performed by use of a functional titration assay as described earlier [22]. PAI-1 activities are given in t-PA inhibitory units using the double chain t-PA standard supplied from the International Committee for Standardization (Holly Hill, England) as a reference. Using this test system, the range of normal values obtained from healthy individuals aged between 20 and 65 years has been found to be 2 to 11 IU/ml [22]. To differentiate between normal and elevated PAI-1 plasma levels we arbitrarily choose the upper 95th percentile of normal values of the healthy controls as a cut-off value (10.7 IU/ml). Depending on the different study designs, blood samples were taken either daily at four different times, or between 06.00 and 09.00 hours to exclude possible influences of the known circadian variations of PAI-1 on the determined plasma levels [23, 24].

Exclusion criteria

Patients with recent signs of inflammatory diseases, with malignancies, and diseases other than CAD associated with thrombosis have been excluded from the study because of possible alterations and consecutive misinterpretations of the results [20, 21, 25].

Results

PAI-1 and the existence of coronary-sclerotic lesions

Although it has been shown by several investigators that PAI-1 is elevated in patients with CAD it has been discussed whether an increased age [18] or recurrent chest pain attacks [19] might be responsible for the results in those patients. Recently published data on PAI-1 and CAD do not compare data of CAD patients with those of age-matched control groups or do not separate patients with stable CAD from such with unstable disease, or do not demonstrate recent angiographic evidence, extent, or exclusion of coronarsclerotic lesions in CAD patients and control individuals. Therefore, interpretation of the results is difficult.

We investigated clinically stable patients (New York Heart Association NYHA Class II; [26]) with angiographically proven CAD and compared the data with those of age-matched patients with a comparable number and intensity of chest-pain attacks but without angiographic evidence of underlying coronary sclerosis. This group (VA) included patients with vasospastic angina [27] or patients with angina-like syndrome without CAD [28]. Thereby a correlation of PAI-1 elevation and coronary sclerosis in age-matched and clinically comparable groups could be shown: about 80 % of the CAD patients but only up to 30 % of the patients without coronary sclerosis (VA) exhibited elevated PAI-1 levels. In patients with valvular disease and in healthy young controls a similar percentage of elevated PAI-1 levels could be shown (Fig. 1) as in patients with vasospastic angina. Furthermore, it was demonstrated that CAD patients with severe coronary sclerosis did not show significantly higher PAI-1 values as compared to CAD patients with moderate sclerotic alterations of coronary arteries. Such a result was also demonstrated by others [17]. In contrast to data recently published [17] we could not demonstrate a significant correlation between PAI-1 levels and elevated plasma triglycerids nor could we demonstrate such correlations with other known risk factors for CAD, e.g., smoking,

60

Table 1. Clinical characteristics of patients with coronary artery disease (CAD), vasospastic angina (VA), valvular disease (VD), and of healthy young volunteers (HV)

	CAD	VA	VD	HV
n	25	15	25	20
m/f	23/2	5/10	11/14	9/11
age	59.8	59.4	58.7	26.5
($\bar{x} \pm$ SD)	±10.2	± 8.7	± 8.2	± 5.1
NYHA II	+	+	−	−
angiographic evidence of coronary sclerosis	+	−	−	n.d.
current risk factors (%)				
smoking	8	0	28	18
hypertension	12	0	4	9
hyperlipidemia (IIb)	56	0	28	0

n.d. = not determined

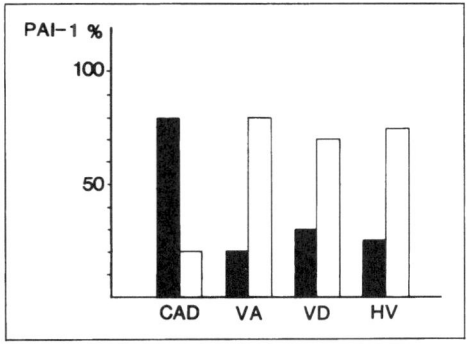

Fig. 1. Percentage of all patients of the respective groups with plasma levels above (■) or below (□) the arbitrarily used cutoff value of 10.7 I.U/ml. CAD = coronary artery disease, VA = vasospastic angina, VD = valvular disease, HV = healthy young volunteers

elevated plasma cholesterol levels, diabetes, or hypertension (data not shown). This lack of correlation might, however, also be due to the relatively small number of patients investigated.

Diurnal fluctuations of PAI-1 plasma levels and onset of acute ischemic attacks

Characteristic diurnal PAI-1 fluctuations are well known and have been described by several authors [23, 24, 29−32]. Highest PAI-1 concentrations have been detected in the early morning hours with an acrophase around 03.00 hours [23, 24]. The combination of PAI-1 elevation and a reduction of the activity of tissue plasminogen activator (tPA) which has been described to exist also in the morning hours [23] might reflect a decrease of the total fibrinolytic potential, and might therefore lead to increased risk for thrombus formation [33]. Clinical studies have shown that the highest incidence of onset of acute myocardial infarctions [34, 35], ischemic attacks [35, 36], and sudden death [37] is between 06.00 and 12.00 hours.

61

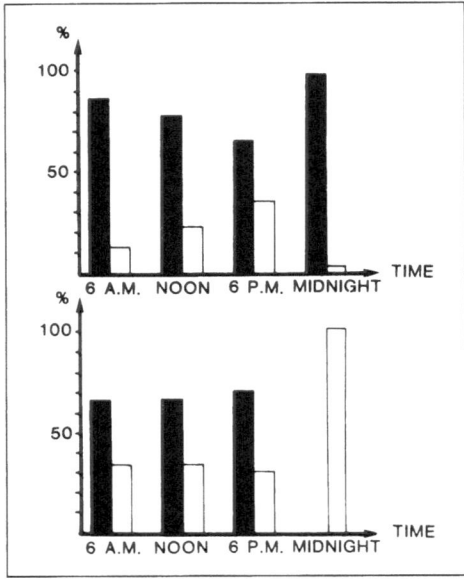

Fig. 2. Percentage of all patients of the respective groups with plasma levels above (■) or below (□) the arbitrarily used cutoff value of 10.7 I.U./ml. The upper panel demonstrates values of patients with acute myocardial infarction. In the lower panel values of patients with unstable angina but without signs of myocardial infarction are shown

We have investigated the diurnal fluctuations of PAI-1 plasma concentrations in patients with unstable angina (NYHA classess III and IV; [26]). Patients included in the study were treated similarly with nitrates (3 mg—6 mg per h i.v.) and a calcium channel blocker (nifedipine, 30 mg — 60 mg per day perorally) but were not treated with heparin and/or inhibitors of platelet aggregation. Blood was taken four times daily (06.00, 12.00, 18.00, 24.00 hours) over a period of at least three days and patients were separated retrospectively into two groups depending on the presence or absence of signs of myocardial infarction. All patients originally presenting with unstable angina exhibited a circadian fluctuation of PAI-1 concentrations with peak values in the early morning [35]. As could be shown further, incidence of severe myocardial ischemia was highest at a median time of 10.00 hours and therefore only some hours after the peak value of PAI-1 [35]. Figure 2 shows the percentages of elevated and normal PAI-1 levels in unstable patients with or without development of myocardial infarction. Patients with myocardial infarction showed a higher percentage of elevated PAI-1 values as compared to the patients group without myocardial infarction. Furthermore, the 24.00 hours PAI-1 levels were significantly more often elevated in the group of myocardial infarction as compared to the respective result in the other group ($p < 0.01$). In the individual patient, onset of ischemic attacks did not alter the typical fluctuation of PAI-1, thereby indicating that PAI-1 elevations in those patients seem not to be induced by chest pain itself [35]. This study does not prove a causal relationship between PAI-1 elevation around 24.00 hours and the peak onset of acute myocardial infarction around 10.00 hours. However, the time relation between these two phenomenons is evident and a causal relationship cannot be generally excluded.

Long-term follow-up of fluctuations of PAI-1 levels and coronary restenosis after successful PTCA

To investigate whether there is a causal relationship between elevation of PAI-1 levels and development of coronary-sclerotic lesions we followed 27 patients who underwent PTCA for one year and determined PAI-1 plasma concentrations one day before and three, six, and 12 months after PTCA. Patients with unsuccessful PTCA were excluded. For the whole observation period clinical course and symptoms were monitored. Objective signs for coronary restenosis were confirmed by coronary arteriography which was performed after six months or earlier if there was evidence of renewed chest pain (Fig. 3). Depending on the angiographically proven development of coronary restenosis patients were separated retrospectively into two groups — one group with, the other group without evidence of coronary restenosis. Ten patients developed coronary restenosis (38 %). Mean age, number of previous myocardial infarctions, extent of coronary artery involvement, site of PTCA, and current risk factors were comparable in both study groups but there was a statistically significant higher number of male patients in the restenosis group as compared to the other group (Table 2). All patients were treated similarly with oral nitrates

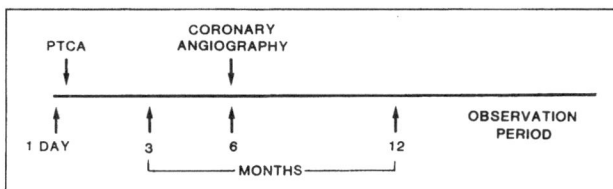

Fig. 3. Time scheme for the follow up study of PAI-1 levels and coronary restenosis in patients after successful PTCA

Table 2. Characteristics of patients with and without coronary restenosis after successful PTCA; MI, myocardial infarction

	Restenosis	No restenosis
n	10	17
m/f	9/1	12/5
age (x ± S.D.)	54.5±1.8	55.8±1.7
previous MI (n)	5	5
number of vessels with stenosis of >70%		
1	5	13
2	3	3
3	2	1
site of PTCA (n)		
LAD	7	11
Cx	1	1
RCA	2	5
risk factors (n)		
smoking	2	3
hypertension	4	7
hyperlipidemia (IIb)	4	7

(5—10 mg isosorbiddinitrate four times daily), calcium channel blockers (30—40 nifedipine daily), and the platelet aggregation inhibitors acetylsalicylic acid (100 mg daily) and dipyridamole (3 × 75 mg daily). As can be seen from Figs. 4A and 4B, patients with development of coronary restenosis showed a smaller decrease of PAI-1 concentrations three and six months after PCTA and furthermore, a significant increase of the mean PAI-1 concentrations after 12 months as compared to patients who did not develop restenosis (p < 0.05).

Following individual variations of PAI-1 concentrations during the observation period in both groups (Figs. 5A and 5B), seven patients of the restenosis group showed a dramatic reincrease of PAI-1 concentrations between three and 12 months after PTCA as compared to an increase of PAI-values in only four of 17 patients in the other group (p < 0.05). Increase of PAI-1 concentration was time-related to the renewed onset of chest pain in five of the seven patients with coronary restenosis.

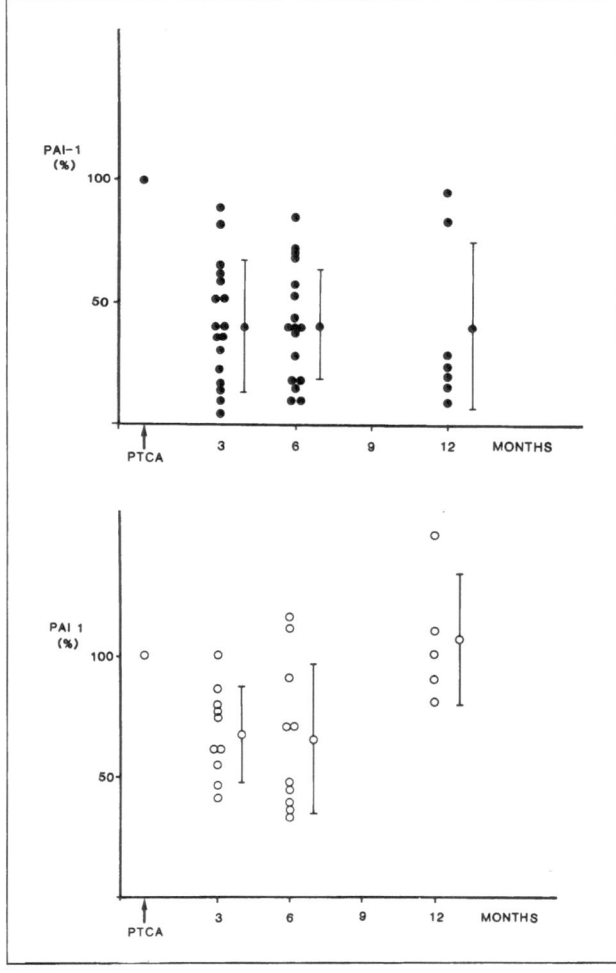

Figs. **4a and b**. Plasma levels of individual patients and their respective means and standard deviations three, six, and 12 months after successful PTCA. Values are given as percentage of the PAI-1 plasma concentrations one day before PTCA. Symbols represent data of patients without (Fig. 4a ●) or with coronary restenosis (Fig. 4b ○)

The remaining two patients had developed coronary restenosis without clinical symptoms.

Conclusions

PAI-1 elevations and the onset of transient ischemic attacks seem to be closely related. The majority of patients with unstable angina and also the majority of patients with clinical evidence of coronary restenosis exhibited onset of chest pain at a time when PAI-1 levels were already increased. However, the results of these studies do not clearly differentiate between onset of PAI-1 increase and renewed onset of ischemic symptoms. This might be due to the low number of time points of blood sam-

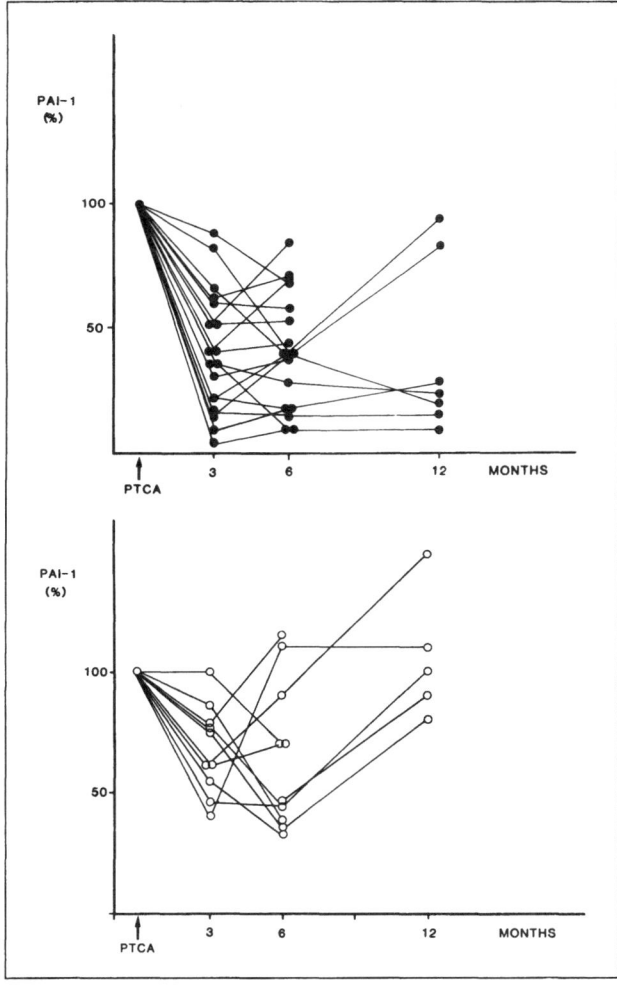

Figs. 5a and b. Individual variations of plasma PAI-1 concentrations in patients without (Fig. 5a ●) or with coronary restenosis (Fig. 5b ○) during the follow-up period. Data are given as percentage of the PAI-1 plasma concentrations one day before PTCA

pling which should be done in shorter intervals. Therefore, results are difficult to interpret. Nevertheless, it might be discussed that in the majority of patients PAI-1 levels seem to indicate the existence of an ongoing coronary-thrombotic process and might therefore be used as a noninvasive marker of coronary thrombus formation. This finding might help to initiate diagnostic and therapeutic measures earlier and therefore lead to a more effective treatment.

References

1. De Wood MA, Spores J, Notske R et al. (1980) Prevalence of total coronary occlusion during the early hours of transmural myocardial infarction. N Engl J Med 303: 897—902
2. Holmes DR, Hartzler GC, Smith HC, Fuster C (1981) Coronary artery thrombosis in patients with unstable angina. Br Heart J 45: 411—416
3. Ganz W, Geft I, Maddahi J et al. (1983) Nonsurgical reperfusion in evolving myocardial infarction. J Am Coll Cardiol, 1: 1247—1253
4. Ganz W, Geft I, Shah P et al. (1984) Intravenous streptokinase in evolving acute myocardial infarction. Am J Cardiol 53: 1209—1216
5. Davis MJ, Thomas A (1984) Thrombosis and acute coronary-artery lesion in sudden cardiac ischemic disease. N Engl J Med 310: 1137—1140
6. Sobel BE, Geltman EM, Tiefenbrunn AJ et al. (1984) Improvement of regional myocardial metabolism after coronary thrombolysis induced with plasminogen activator or streptokinase. Circulation 69: 983—990
7. Falk E (1985) Unstable angina with fatal outcome: dynamic coronary thrombosis leading to infarction and/or sudden death. Circulation 71: 699—708
8. Stehbens WE (1985) Relationship of coronary artery thrombosis to myocardial infarction. Lancet 2: 639—642
9. Fuster V, Badimon L, Ambrose JA, Turitto V, Badimon JJ, Adams PC, Chesebro JH (1987) Pathogenetic and angiographic features in unstable angina and other coronary syndromes. Thromb Haemostas 58: 246 (abstract 911)
10. Higashino Y, Katoh O, Rakugi H, Tateyama H, Suzuki K, Minamino T (1987) Angiographic morphology in unstable angina — serial changes from acute to chronic stage. Circulation 76 (Suppl.) IV, 451 (abstract 1797)
11. Estelles A, Tormo G, Azar J, Espana F, Tormo V (1985) Reduced fibrinolytic activity in coronary heart disease in basal conditions and after exercise. Thromb Res 40: 373—383
12. Hamsten A, Witman B, De Faire U, Blombäck M (1985) Increased plasma levels of rapid inhibitor of tissue plasminogen activator in young survivors of myocardial infarction. N Engl J Med 313: 1557—1563
13. Hamsten A, Blombäck M, Witman B et al. (1986) Haemostatic function in myocardial infarction. Br Heart J 55: 58—66
14. Paramo JA, Colucci M, Collen D (1985) Plasminogen activator inhibitor in the blood of patients with coronary artery disease. Br Med J 291: 574—575
15. Huber K, Resch I, Rosc D, Lang I, Stefenelli Th, Glogar DH, Binder BR (1987) Plasminogen-activator-Inhibitor-Plasmaspiegel bei koronarer Herzkrankheit, vasospastischer Angina und Herzklappenerkrankungen. Z Kardiol 76: 36 (abstract 96)
16. Korninger C, Jäger R, Huber K, Lechner K (1988) Levels of plasminogen activator inhibitor levels in coronary artery disease: correlation with age and serum triglyceride concentrations. J Am Coll Cardiol 9: 263—268
17. Mehta J, Mehta P, Lawson D, Saldeen T. Plasma tissue plasminogen activator inhibitior levels in coronary artery disease: correlation with age and serum triglyceride concentrations. J Am Coll Cardiol 1987; 9, 263—68.
18. Hashimoto Y, Kobayashi A, Yamazuki N, Sugawara Y, Takada Y, Takada A (1987) Relationship between age and plasma t-PA, PA inhibitor and PA activity. Thromb Res 1987; 46: 625—633
19. Gram J, Kluft C, Jespersen J (1987) Depression of tissue plasminogen activator (t-PA) activity and rise of t-PA inhibition and acute phase reactants in blood of patients with acute myocardial infarction (AMI). Thromb Haemostas 58: 817—821

20. Juhan-Vague I, Aillaud MF, De Cock F, Philip-Joet C, Arnaud C, Serradimigni A, Collen D (1985) The fast-acting inhibitor of tissue-type plasminogen activator is an acute phase reactant protein. In: Progress in Fibrinolysis. Davidson JF, Donati MB, Coccheri S (eds.) Vol. VII, pp. 146—149, Churchill Livingstone, Edinburgh — London—Melbourne—New York
21. Kruithof EKO, Gudinchet A, Bachmann F (1988) Plasminogen activator inhibitor 1 and plasminogen activator inhibitor 2 in various disease states. Thromb Haemostas — in press
22. Korninger C, Wagner O, Binder BR (1985) Tissue plasminogen activator inhibitor in human plasma: development of a functional assay system and demonstration of a correlating M_r 50,000 antiactivator. J Lab Clin Med 105: 718—724
23. Andreotti F, Davies GJ, Hackett D, Khan MI, De Dart A, Dooijewaard G, Maseri A, Kluft C (1988) Circadian variation of fibrinolytic factors in normal human plasma. Fibrinolysis 2: 90—92
24. Huber K, Beckmann R, Lang I, Schuster E, Binder BR (1988) Circadian fluctuations in plasma levels of tissue plasminogen activator antigen and plasminogen activator inhibitor activity. Fibrinolysis — in press
25. Juhan-Vague I, Valadier J, Alessi MC, Aillaud MF, Ansaldi J, Philip-Joet C, Holvoet P, Serradimigni A, Collen D (1987) Deficient t-PA release and elevated PA inhibitor levels in patients with spontaneous or recurrent deep venous thrombosis. Thromb Haemostas 57: 67—72
26. The Criteria Committee of New York Heart Association (1964). In: Diseases of the heart and blood vessels; nomenclature and criteria for diagnosis, ed. 6, Little Brown, New York
27. Heupler FA, Proudfit WL, Razavi M, Shirey EK, Greenstreet R, Sheldon WC (1978) Ergonovine maleate provocative test for coronary arterial spasm. Am J Cardiol 41: 631—640
28. Pasternak RC, Thibault GE, Savoia M, De Sanctis RW, Huter AM Jr (1980) Chest pain with angiographically insignificant coronary arterial obstruction. Clinical presentation and long-term follow up. Am J Med 68: 813—819
29. Fearnley GR, Balmforth G, Fearnley E (1957) Evidence of a diurnal fibrinolytic rhythm; with a simple method of measuring natural fibrinolysis. Clin Sci 16: 645—650
30. Rosing DR, Brakman P, Redwood DR, Goldstein RE, Beiser GD, Astrup T, Epstein SE (1970) Blood fibrinolytic activity in man. Diurnal variation and the response to varying intensities of exercise. Circ Res 27: 171—184
31. Cepelak V, Barcal R, Cepelakova H, Mayer O. (1978) Circadian rhythm of fibrinolysis. In: Davidson JF, Rowan RM, Samama MM, Desnoyer PC (eds) Progress in Chemical Fibrinolysis and Thrombolysis, Vol. 3, Raven Press, New York 571—578
32. Kluft C (1978) C1-inactivator-resistant fibrinolytic activity in plasma euglobulin fractions: its relation to vascular activator in blood and its role in euglobulin fibrinolysis. Thromb Res 13: 135—151
33. Bachmann F (1987) Fibrinolysis. In: Verstraete M, Vermylen J, Lijnen R, Arnout J (eds) Thrombosis and Haemostasis 1987, Leuven University Press, pp. 227—265
34. Muller JA, Stone PH, Turi ZG et al (1985) Circadian variation in the frequency of onset of acute myocardial infarction. N Eng J Med 313: 1315—1322
35. Huber K, Rosc D, Resch I, Schuster E, Glogar DH, Binder BR (1988) Circadian fluctuations of plasminogen activator inhibitor and tissue plasminogen activator levels in plasma of patients with unstable coronary artery disease and acute myocardial infarction. Thromb Haemostas — in press
36. Rocco MB, Barry J, Campbell S et al (1987) Circadian variation of transient myocardial ischemia in patients with coronary artery disease. Circulation 75: 375—400
37. Muller JA, Ludmer PL, Willich SN et al. (1987) Circadian variation in the frequency of sudden cardiac death. Circulation 75: 131—138

Author's address:
Dr. Kurt Huber
Kardiologische Univ. Klinik
Garnisongasse 13
A-1090 Wien
Austria

Discussion

MASERI:

Were your patients on aspirin?

HUBER:

They were on 100 mg of aspirin a day.

PATRONO:

Is there any possibility to influence the level of PAI-1, and what about a long treatment with N3 fatty acids?

HUBER:

I do not know about the long-term treatment with this fatty acid, especially in our patients. We conducted a pilot study to see if there are effects from taking nitrates, taking calcium channel blockers, taking aspirin or dipyridamole, and there was no effect on the PAI-1 plasma levels.

KRUCOFF:

We have heard two different aspects of PAI-1. One is a part of a pathway that may be involved in the pathogenesis of the disease and its changing to an acute form. The other is a basic marker of progression of the disease. I wonder if you would comment on how your dta supports each of these? Especially abount the role of PAI-1 in the pathogenesis of the disease and whether or not PAI-1 in fact is a marker that should be followed or should be used as a reason for further survey.

HUBER:

I can only hypothesize in answer to these two questions. First, the relationship between elevated PAI-1 levels and thromboembolic complications or coronary thrombus formation. I think we can only show this interesting time-relation in patients, in normals, and in patients with high PAI-1 levels in the morning hours and we might suspect that during that time when on the other hand TPA activities are low, there may be a higher risk for thrombus-formation and I believe that some hours of high risk of thrombus-formation might be enough to form a clot that is strong enough to occlude a vessel. But this is only a hypothesis.

About restenosis, we originally thought that we would find more early re-increase in PAI-1 levels in patients before they were symptomatic. That we did not find this result might depend on the relatively long interval of three months between the blood collections. We performed regular blood collections every day one week after successful PTCA and within this one week we did not see a decrease of the PAI-1 levels as compared to the pre-PTCA value. The decrease that has been shown in almost all patients must become evident after some weeks and not very early, but it is, from our data, not clear whether PAI-1 levels really re-increase before there is a sign for symptoms of restenosis. That is why we say this might be a noninvasive marker because in almost all patients with a re-increase of PAI-1 levels you find an ongoing coronary thrombotic process.

ANDREOTTI:

Did you correlate the number of vessel disease involvement and the levels of triglyceride with the PAI-1 levels in the first group of patients that you studied?

HUBER:

Well, we find a very weak correlation between elevated triglycerides and PAI-1 levels. If you compare patients with one-, two-, three-vessel disease, there is obviously no difference in the PAI-1 concentrations. This might be an indirect sign that a more acute problem, if it is only in one vessel, is responsible for elevated PAI-1.

ANDREOTTI:

How would you explain the increased PAI-1 levels before PTCA?

HUBER:

Most of these patients had a partially unstable coronary artery disease and about 40% were not unstable but they had high grade stenosis, so we find elevated PAI-1 levels in almost all patients with coronary artery disease. This might be the explanation for this finding.

ANDREOTTI:

I would like to make two comments in response to one question. How is it possible to modulate PAI-1 levels in plasma? There are two pharmaceutical ways of lowering PAI-1 levels: Oral contraceptives is one, anabolic steriods is another. The other comment on PAI-1 and the recurrence of myocardial infarction which has been shown in two studies, one by Harmsten and another by Kram, both statistically shows a high level PAI-1 or a reduction of fibrinolytic activity in those that have a recurrence of myocardial infarction.

GOHLKE:

How do you explain the decrease of PAI-1 after PTCA?

HUBER:

My explanation is that PAI-1 levels are more often elevated if there is an ongoing thrombotic process after PTCA. In most of these patients you have a good result, and I think you have no problem of recurrence. There are obviously no significant stenoses after PTCA and I think this might be the explanation.

Platelet activation in unstable angina

C. Patrono, and M. Vejar

Department of Pharmacology, Catholic University School of Medicine, Rome, Italy, and Cardiovascular Unit, Royal Postgraduate Medical School, London, UK

Introduction

Coronary thrombi range in size from focal aggregates of platelets detectable by scanning electron microscopy only, to a mass large enough to occlude a major coronary artery. The former are probably very common in all subjects who have advanced atheroma [1]. Thrombi large enough to produce clinical symptoms directly by altering blood flow can be detected angiographically and/or angioscopically, and in necropsy studies they can be reconstructed from serial histological sections to assess the structure of underlying intima to elucidate factors which initiate thrombosis [1]. These reconstructions show that both deep and superficial intimal injury can invoke thombus formation. The latter is associated with endothelial loss ("denudation injury") with exposure of the immediately underlying connective tissue matrix [1]. Deep intimal injury underlies 75 % of large intraluminal thrombi and is the results of tears or splits extending deep into the intima from the lumen [1]. Plaque fissures with overlying mural thrombi are the morphological basis of angiographic type II lesions, described both in patients with unstable angina [2] and following thrombolysis in acute myocardial infarction [3].

Evidence for episodic platelet activation and thrombosis in unstable angina

The results of two independent studies have demonstrated the prevalence of recurrent mural thrombosis in a major epicardial artery with peripheral embolization in patients with unstable angina suffering sudden ischemic cardiac death [4, 5].

In the study of Falk [4], 81 % of the coronary thrombi were found to have a layered structure with thrombus material of differing ages, which indicates that they were formed successively by repeated mural deposits which progressed to total vascular occlusion in an episodic way. This recurrent thrombus formation was accompanied by intermittent fragmentation in 73 % of the cases, with peripheral embolization causing micro-embolic occlusion of small intramyocardial arteries associated with micro-infarcts. In this series of 22 patients, the frequency with which platelet emboli were found in patients with unstable angina (53 %) was higher than that in patients without unstable angina (43 %), but the difference did not reach statistical significance [4]. In contrast, in the larger series of Davies et al. [5], intramyocardial platelet emboli were found with a significantly higher incidence in patients who had unstable angina (44.4 %) than in those who did not (20.4 %). The majority of platelet aggregates had either a minimal or no fibrin component and were found in vessels ranging in size from precapillary arterioles to arteries 1 mm in diameter [5].

The results of recent angiographic [2] and angioscopic [6] studies largely confirm both the nature and specificity of coronary lesions in unstable angina.

Reliable assessment of platelet activation in vivo, based on measurements of platelet-derived products (e.g., PF_4, βTG, TXB_2) in peripheral and/or coronary sinus blood, has been hampered by methodological as well as analytical problems [7]. The former are related to substantial ex vivo platelet activation occurring both during and after sampling; the latter probably reflect significant cross-reactivities of long-lived enzymatic metabolites of TXB_2 with antisera raised against the parent compound. Thus, as little as 0.1 % of maximal platelet activation ex vivo is sufficient to generate apparent "circulating" concentrations of TXB_2 on the order of 200—300 pg/ml [8]. On the other hand, most anti-TXB_2 sera very effectively (i. e., by 50—100 %) recognize 2,3-dinor-TXB_2 which has a plasma half-life at least twice as long as that of TXB_2 [9].

An alternative approach based on measurement of the urinary excretion of the major enzymatic derivatives of TXB_2 was proposed to circumvent the above problems [10, 11]. Thus, Fitzgerald et al. [10] reported sporadic increases in the urinary excretion of 2,3-dinor-TXB_2 in 16 patients with unstable angina in relation to episodes of chest pain. In contrast, metabolite excretion was normal in patients with stable coronary disease, both at rest and after excercise-induced myocardial ischemia [10]. Vejar et al. [11] measured the urinary excretion of 11-dehydro-TXB_2 in 21 patients with unstable angina in relation to clinical and/or ECG changes. The latter metabolite is at least as abundant a conversion product of exogenously infused TXB_2 as 2,3-dinor-TXB_2 [12], previously characterized as the most abundant urinary metabolite of TXB_2 in man [13]. Twenty-five of 56 (i. e., 45 %) 6—8 h urine samples obtained from patients with unstable angina showed increased (> 2SD of controls) 11-dehydro-TXB_2 excretion, during treatment with iv isosorbide dinitrate and oral diltiazem. Of these, only three episodes of enhanced metabolite excretion were associated with ST-segment changes, seven with chest pain and 15 with no ECG or clinical changes [11]. Although somewhat at variance in relating biochemical evidence of platelet activation to the occurrence of spontaneous myocardial ischemia, the results of Fitzgerald et al. [10] and of Vejar et al. [11] concur in establishing the following features of platelet activation in unstable angina: a) the biosynthetic capacity of platelets to generate TXB_2, when maximally stimulated ex vivo, is unchanged; b) the metabolic disposition of endogenously released TXB_2, through β-oxidation and 11-OH-dehydrogenation, is substantially unaltered; c) enhanced TXB_2 production occurs episodically in the vast majority of patients, though the number of such episodes is greatly variable among patients.

Evidence for a local thrombotic process as a dominant alteration

The results of the post-mortem studies quoted above are also in agreement: platelet masses are confined to segments of myocardium downstream of an atheromatous plaque over which thrombus has developed [4, 5]. Moreover, both studies show that multifocal microscopic necrosis is closely associated with the presence of platelet emboli. Such a selective distribution of platelet aggregates in the microcirculation distal to thrombosed epicardial arteries would argue against a systemic cause, such as "hyperreactive" platelets, underlying spontaneous intravascular agglutination in the microvascular bed. In contrast, these findings are highly suggestive of localized platelet aggregation occurring repeatedly in a major coronary artery as a result of plaque fissure, exposing platelets to lipids and collagen of the ruptured intimal cap. The results of biochemical measurements [10, 11] are consistent with this hypothesis.

Davies et al. [5] suggested that platelet emboli in the myocardium may cause symptoms by release of pharmacologically active substances such as TXA_2 and serotonin, which increase vasomotor tone to a degree similar to that induced by the physical plugging of small vessels. However, the 44 % incidence of platelet aggregates in patients with chest pain of recent onset reported in this study clearly indicates that more than 50 % of patients had unstable angina unrelated to intramyocardial platelet emboli. On the other hand, the 20 % incidence in patients without a history of unstable angina suggests that the presence of platelet aggregates in the myocardium does not necessarily evoke anginal symptoms. Moreover, Vejar et al. [11] recently demonstrated dissociation of platelet activation, as reflected by enhanced excretion of 11-dehydro-TXB_2, and spontaneous myocardial ischemia, as monitored by 24-h Holter. Thus, although the two events may represent functional expressions of the same coronary lesion, they are likely to be triggered by independent mechanisms through different mediators.

Can intracoronary platelet aggregation be prevented?

The role of aspirin in the prevention of coronary thrombosis was reviewed recently [14]. A Veterans Administration Cooperative Study [15] demonstrated that a single daily administration of aspirin 324 mg in buffered solution, started within 51 h of admission to the hospital, significantly reduced the 12-week incidence of acute myocardial infarction or death by 51 % in men with unstable angina. These results have been substantially confirmed by a Canadian Multicenter Trial in patients of both sexes treated with aspirin 325 mg qid [16]. The rate of death or acute myocardial infarction was also found to be 51 % lower in the group treated with aspirin, after a mean follow-up period of 18 months [16]. To put these figures into perspective, one should consider that, given a 12—14 % event rate at one year, treatment of 100 patients with aspirin will protect 6—7 patients from a non-fatal myocardial infarction or cardiac death. Despite the surprisingly identical figures of risk reduction in the two trials, there are a number of important differences in design and in several patient-or drug-related variables that should be taken into account when comparing the two studies. Some of the major differences are outlined in Table 1.

Aspirin inhibits TXA_2-dependent platelet function by irreversibly acetylating platelet cyclooxygenase, the enzyme that converts arachidonate released from membrane phospholipids into prostaglandin (PG) endoperoxides [17]. Besides being a potent inducer of irreversible platelet aggregation, TXA_2 also constricts vascular smooth muscle including human coronary artery [17]. Thus, the beneficial effects of aspirin in unstable angina might be theoretically related to prevention of platelet

Table 1. Variables in the aspirin trials in unstable angina.

	V.A. Cooperative Study (15)	Canadian Multicenter Trial (16)
Start	1974	1979
Number of patients	1266 (2 groups)	555 (4 groups)
Unstable angina patients entered	18.3%	11.7%
Interval between CCU admission and randomization	51 hours	192 hours
Sex	Male	Male & Female (27%)
Duration of treatment	12 weeks	104 weeks
ASA dosage	324 mg/day	325 mg qid
Beta-blockers	74% (at some time) 42% (all the time)	80% at entry
Calcium-antagonists	?	30% at entry
CABG	3.5%	31.5%
Reduction of cardiac death or MI		
by efficacy analysis	51% (P = 0.0005)	51% (P = 0.008)
by intention to treat	41% (P = 0.004)	30% (P = 0.072)
	[patients with MI at entry (n = 72) included in the analysis]	(patients with MI excluded from trial)

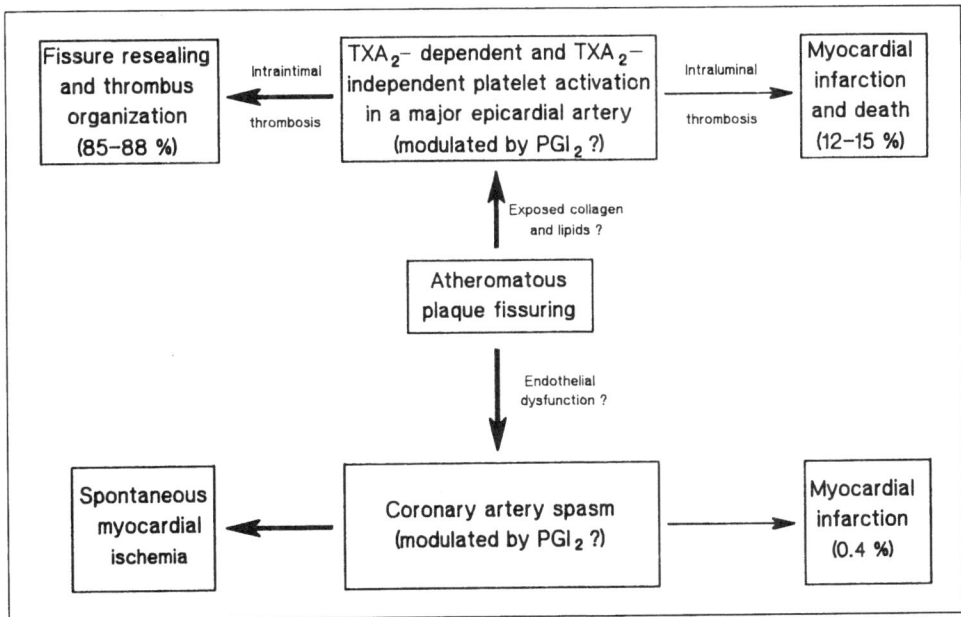

Fig. 1. Interplay of plaque fissuring, intracoronary platelet activation, and hyperreactivity of a segment of vascular smooth muscle in unstable angina. (The contribution and interplay of different mechanisms are discussed in the text and, in greater detail, in [21, 22].)

aggregation and subsequent vascular occlusion and/or to prevention of coronary vasospasm. The latter possibility, however, is contradicted by the failure of aspirin to prevent acute myocardial ischemia due to coronary vasospasm in patients with variant angina [18], and by the unchanged incidence or severity of angina in the aspirin-treated patients studied by the Veterans Administration Cooperative Study [19]. These observations are consistent with the lack of an important causal link between episodic platelet activation and spontaneous myocardial ischemia [11], as discussed above. Thus, suppression of TXA_2-mediated platelet aggregation seems a more likely mechanism to account for the reported benefit of aspirin in the latter study, but this does not exclude other explanations. This interpretation is further strengthened by the fact that these beneficial effects were demonstrated in association with a single daily administration of the drug. Given the short half-life (20—30 minutes) of intact acetylsalicylic acid in the human circulation, these results are consistent with permanent inactivation by aspirin of an enzyme or receptor that cannot be resynthesised to a critical level within the 24-h interval between dosing. Acetylation of platelet cyclooxygenase might represent such an irreversible process, although the dose of aspirin used (324 mg) does not allow the exclusion of other acetylation processes because it is 8—10 times in excess of the amount needed to fully inhibit platelet TXA_2 production during chronic dosing [20].

Conclusion

Figure 1 attempts to relate intracoronary platelet activation to plaque fissuring and to "hyperreactivity" of coronary smooth muscle [21, 22], on the basis of different pieces of information that were reviewed in this paper: a) necropsy reconstructions of events occurring in those patients with unstable angina who died [4, 5]; b) short-term (2—5 days) biochemical and functional measurements performed in patients undergoing various pharmacological treatments during the unstable phase [10, 11]; c) controlled clinical trials of antiplatelet therapy with aspirin, initiated within 2 to 8 days after admission and continued for 12 to 104 weeks [15, 16]. Each of the above approaches suffers from limitations inherent to the nature of the investigation and each looks at different subsets of patients within a variable time-frame. Despite this, they are coherent in relating a rather specific pattern of episodic platelet activation to a localized coronary event, i.e., rupture or fissuring of an atheromatous plaque. Moreover, they indicate that TXA_2-dependent platelet activation plays an important role in the progression towards complete coronary occlusion, that occurs in approximately 10 % to 15 % of all patients who underwent an unstable phase. The fact that a substantial proportion of myocardial infarctions and deaths do occur despite aspirin therapy (see Table 1) would suggest that TXA_2-independent platelet aggregation in a major epicardial coronary artery may be responsible for such events. Finally, episodic platelet activation is infrequently associated with spontaneous myocardial ischemia [11] and the latter does not appear to benefit from antiplatelet therapy [19]. At variance with previous suggestions [5, 10], we would like to propose that platelet activation and spontaneous myocardial ischemia may reflect different aspects of the same lesion, such as exposure of platelets to lipids and collagen of the ruptured intimal cap and endothelial dysfunction, respectively, and be triggered by

74

independent mechanisms through different mediators [11]. Whether a substantial sparing of endothelial PGI_2 production in the immediate vicinity of a fissured plaque might favorably affect its clinical expression (in terms of altered vasomotion) and/or its thrombotic evolution (in terms of TXA_2-independent pathways of platelet aggregation) remains to be established. Both selective inhibitors of platelet TXA_2 synthesis (e.g., low-dose aspirin, TX-synthase inhibitors) and antagonists of PGH_2/TXA_2 receptors are now available to test this challenging hypothesis.

Acknowledgments

The expert editorial assistance of Maria Luisa Bonanomi and Egidio Diaferia is gratefully acknowledged. The studies of the authors were supported by grants from the British Heart Foundation, the British Council, and the Italian National Research Council (CNR, Progetto Finalizzato Medicina Preventiva e Riabilitativa: 86.01894.56 and 87.00398.56).

References

1. Davies MJ (1988) The role of platelets in vascular obstruction in coronary artery disease. In: FitzGerald GA, Patrono C (eds) Platelets and Vascular Occlusion. Raven Press, New York (in press)
2. Ambrose JA, Winters, SL, Arora RR, Haft JI, Goldstein J, Rentrop KP, Gorlin R, Fuster V (1985) Angiographic morphology in myocardial infarction. A link between the pathogenesis of unstable angina and myocardial infarction. J Am Coll Cardiol 6: 1233—1238
3. Ambrose JA, Winters SL, Arora RR, Eng A, Riccio A, Gorlin R, Fuster V (1986) Angiographic evolution of coronary artery morphology in unstable angina. J Am Coll Cardiol 7: 472—478
4. Falk E (1985) Unstable angina with fatal outcome: dynamic coronary thrombosis leading to infarction and/or sudden death. Circulation 71: 699—708
5. Davies MJ, Thomas AC, Knapman PA, Hangartner JR (1986) Intramyocardial platelet aggregation in patients with unstable angina suffering sudden ischaemic cardiac death. Circulation 73: 418—427
6. Sherman CT, Litvack F, Grundfest W, Lee ME, Hickey A, Chaux A, Kass R, Blanche C, Morgenstern L, Ganz W, Swan HJC, Matloff J, Forrester JS (1986) Coronary angioscopy in patients with unstable angina pectoris. N Engl J Med 315: 913—919
7. FitzGerald GA, Pedersen AK, Patrono C (1983) Analysis of prostacyclin and thromboxane biosynthesis in cardiovascular disease. Circulation 67: 1174-1177
8. Patrono C, Ciabattoni G, Pugliese F, Pierucci A, Blair IA, FitzGerald GA (1986) Estimated rate of thromboxane secretion into the circulation of normal humans. J Clin Invest 77: 590—594
9. Lawson JA, Patrono C, Ciabattoni G, FitzGerald GA (1986) Long-lived enzymatic metabolites of thromboxane B_2 in the human circulation. Analyt Biochem 155: 198—205
10. Fitzgerald DJ, Roy L, Catella F, FitzGerald GA (1986) Platelet activation in unstable coronary disease. N Engl J Med 315: 983—989
11. Vejar M, Lipkin DP, Maseri A, Born GVR, Ciabattoni G, Patrono C (1988) Dissociation of platelet activation and spontaneous myocardial ischemia in unstable angina. Clin Res 36: 326A
12. Ciabattoni G, Pugliese F, Davi G, Pierucci A, Simonetti BM, Patrono C (1988) Fractional conversion of thromboxane B_2 to urinary 11-dehydro-thromboxane B_2 in man. Submitted for publication.
13. Roberts LJ II, Sweetman BJ, Oates JA (1981) Metabolism of thromboxane B_2 in man. Identification of twenty urinary metabolites. J Biol Chem 256: 8384—8393
14. Patrono C (1986) Aspirin for the prevention of coronary thrombosis: current facts and perspectives. Eur Heart J 7: 454—459

15. Lewis HD Jr, Davis JW, Archibald DG, Steinke WE, Smitherman TC, Doherty JE, Schnaper HW, Le Winter MM, Linares E, Pouget JM, Sabharwal SC, Chesler E, De Mots H (1983) Protective effects of aspirin against acute myocardial infarction and death in men with unstable angina. Results of a Veterans Administration Cooperative Study. N Engl J Med 309: 396—403

16. Cairns JA, Gent M, Singer J, Finnie KJ, Froggatt GM, Holder DA, Jablonsky G, Kostuk WJ, Melendez LJ, Myers MG, Sackett DL, Sealey BJ, Transer PH (1985) Aspirin, sulfinpyrazone, or both in unstable angina. Results of a Canadian Multicenter Trial. N Engl J Med 313: 1369—1375

17. Majerus PW (1983) Arachidonate metabolism in vascular disorders. J. Clin Invest 72: 1521—1525

18. Chierchia S, De Caterina R, Crea F, Patrono C, Maseri A (1982) Failure of thromboxane A_2 blockade to prevent attacks of vasospastic angina. Circulation 66: 702—705

19. Lewis HD Jr, Davis JW, Archibald DG (1984) Letter to the editor. N Engl J Med 310: 122

20. Patrono C, Ciabattoni G, Patrignani P, Pugliese F, Filabozzi P, Catella F, Davì G, Forni L (1985) Clinical pharmacology of platelet cyclooxygenase inhibition. Circulation 72: 1177—1184

21. Maseri A, Chierchia S, Davies G (1986) Pathophysiology of coronary occlusion in acute infarction. Circulation 73: 233—239

22. Chierchia S, Patrono C (1987) Role of platelet and vascular eicosanoids in the pathophysiology of ischemic heart disease. Federation Proc 46: 81—88

Authors' address:
Professor Carlo Patrono
Istituto di Farmacologia
Università Cattolica del Sacro Cuore
Largo F. Vito 1
00168 Rome, Italy

Discussion

KUPPER:

I have a question about your PTCA patients with the elevated TXB_2 metabolite excretion in urine. Could you by chance analyze one patient where the PTCA instrumentarium was inserted but no PTCA carried out?

PATRONO:

We do have one such patient, and he does show some increase by 50% to 60%, but nothing compared to the kind of multifold increases in metabolite excretion that we found in those who actually had two to six dilatations.

CHIERCHIA:

I only partially agree with the first of your conclusions, that platelet reactivation is only partially or not related with ischemic events. You take the evidence for that statement from the fact that there was no relationship between episodic increases in TX activity, as opposed to ST segment depression and angina. I think there are two points to take into account. One is the temporal resolution of your urinary sampling, which is after all only eight hours. So you cannot establish a firm temporal relationship between the two. And second, the methodological problem is that pain certainly, and ECG as well, are very crude indicators of myocardial ischemia. So you cannot rule out an association between thrombotic activity and ischemia purely on the absence of significant ST segment depression on the ECG.

PATRONO:

I take your point. On the other hand, such a relationship was suggested on much weaker grounds. That is, it was suggested by a study where metabolite excretion was related to episodes of chest pain, forget about the ECG. And although it is difficult to argue with what you say, I think one additional point which is consistent with such a lack of close association is the lack of an effect of drugs wich interfere with platelet activation on the occurrence of myocardial ischemia. I mean, if the two are temporally and causally related, then one would expect to see an effect of drugs affecting thromboxin production on the occurrence of myocardial ischemia, which as you know is not the case.

DE CATERINA:

What is your hypothesis to explain the lack of elevation of this metabolite in peripheral arterial disease as opposed to unstable angina? There have been reports that platelet activation occurs in this desease, and actually there is some pathological background to postulate that active or erupted placques may exist in the circulation of these patients, so you would expect some degree of platelet activation — could this bring your levels up?

PATRONO:

It might be related to the extent of the diffusion of the disease. The only really reliable data that exist in the literature were obtained in patients with very severe diffuse arterio sclerotic disease who were diabetic. These are the only ones that I know of. There are of course hundreds of papers which base the evidence for increased platelet thromboxin production or increased aggregation on ex vivo measurement, but I think that those are hopeless in terms of possible interpretation.

ANDREOTTI:

You showed us that the secretion rate of thromboxin metabolites in urine in arteriosclerotic patients with chronic stable angina was constant over the 24 h. Do you feel that this is in contradiction to the reported morning increase of platelet aggregability in normals and patients with coronary artery disease?

PATRONO:

They were obviously not the same kind of patients, but as I said in the beginning, these are measurements of a different nature. On the one hand you are looking at what happens in vivo, what happens in terms of actual production of this substance. On the other hand, when you look at platelet aggregation ex vivo, you are looking at a capacity index, and depending on the condition of the aggregation assay you can say whatever you like, I mean depending on whether you study platelet aggregation response to one stimulus, or two, or three, and there are reasons for doing all these kinds of things, depending upon the concentration of the stimulus, you can say that the platelets are hyperreactive or hyperaggregable, but as I tried to point out, you do not really need to have hyper-aggregable platelets to have a valid reason for what Prof. Davis sees at autopsy findings.

ANDREOTTI:

So you would not exclude that platelet aggregation in vivo does not show a circadian pattern?

PATRONO:

I do not exclude that that is the case. I only tend to say that, a) we do not know what it means, do not know what platelet aggregation ex vivo means in terms of what happens in vivo, and b) I think that we do not need to have that in order to account for what happens.

Prostaglandin metabolites in unstable angina pectoris patients

W. Kupper, C. W. Hamm, W. Bleifeld

Department of Cardiology, Medical Clinic, University Hospital Eppendorf, Hamburg, FRG

Introduction

Thromboxane A_2 is the principle metabolite of arachidonic acid in platelets. It stimulates platelet activation and is hydrolyzed rapidly (half-life time of 30s) to the inactive product thromboxane B_2.

Prostacyclin, mainly synthetized in endothelial cells, potently inhibits the aggregation of platelets; its biologically inactive hydration product is 6-keto-prostaglandin F_1alpha.

The measurement of plasma concentrations of thromboxane B_2 or 6-keto-prostaglandin F_1alpha is of little value as an index of their production in vivo. Much of the published information on prostaglandin formation in humans has been confounded by methodological problems or artificial prostaglandin formation or both [2, 5, 9, 12].

The analysis of urinary metabolites represents a non-invasive but indirect approach to the assessment of prostanoid formation in vivo and can be taken as an index of the total body production of prostanoids. Clearly, one cannot specifically attribute a tissue of origin to the material measured. On the other hand, any phasic release pattern of thromboxane A_2 or prostacyclin may not escape detection.

The key pathogenetic role of platelets and their constituents in the pathogenesis of unstable angina is supported by angiographic [1, 3, 8, 16] (Fig. 1), angioscopic, [13], and autopsy proofs [4].

In our study we investigated whether platelet activation in vivo is detectable by means of 2.3-dinor-thromboxane B_2 urinary excretion in patients with unstable angina. Furthermore, we tested the hypothesis of a reduced prostacycline formation.

Patients and methods

Patients were classified according to the clinical course of the unstable phase. Sixteen patients (three female, 13 male; mean age 66 ± 9 years) with more than a 15 min-duration angina of new onset or of abruptly increasing intensity represented the unstable angina group. On the basis of the duration of intravenous nitroglycerine infusion after admission, two subgroups were formed. Ten patients could not be stabilized despite aggressive medical treatment that included intravenous nitroglycerine for more than 48 h, calcium channel antagonists, and betareceptor blockers; they were classified as "non-responders". The remaining six patients responded well

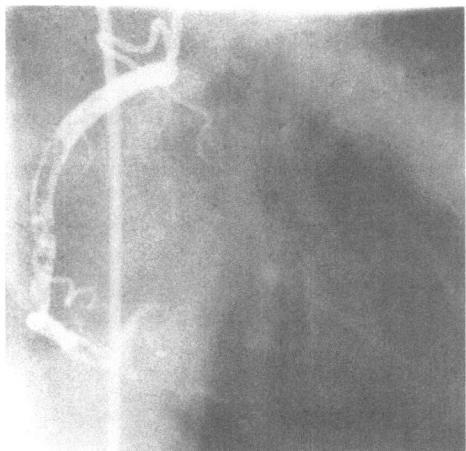

Fig. 1. Large intraluminal filling defect as a sign of intracoronary thrombus in the mid position of the right coronary artery.

to intravenous nitroglycerine and were symptom-free after a mean duration of intravenous nitroglycerine of 17 ± 23 h; they were classified as "responders".

Eight patients (one female, seven male; mean age 49 ± 8 years) had sustained postinfarction angina at rest without clinical evidence of postinfarction pericarditis built the postinfarction angina group.

Protocol

In each patient, urine was collected in three consecutive 8-h-periods before or after an interval of at least 48 h following cardiac catheterization. During the collection of urine, continuous two-lead ambulatory ECG monitoring was performed (Medilog MR 14, Oxford Instruments) with electrodes placed in the lead V2 and V5 positions. Not evaluated were patients with a history of typical variant angina or intake of acetylsalicylic acid, sulfine pyrazone, indomethacine, or related non-steroidal anti-inflammatory drugs within the last two weeks.

Coronary angiography was performed in the mean after three to four days following admission. Evidence of a thrombus was defined as an intraluminal filling defect, circumferentially outlined by contrast medium or hazy intracoronary staining and stasis of contrast medium at the site of a coronary stenosis.

Chemical analysis

Analysis of the urine samples was performed without knowledge of clinical data (Prof. P. C. Weber, Med. Klinik Innenstadt, Munich, FRG). Assay of urinary 2,3-dinor-thromboxane B_2 was performed by high performance liquid chromatography and radioimmunoassay, assay of urinary 2,3-dinor-6-keto prostaglandin F_1alpha was performed by combined gaschromatography mass spectrometry monitoring ion pairs as previously described [7].

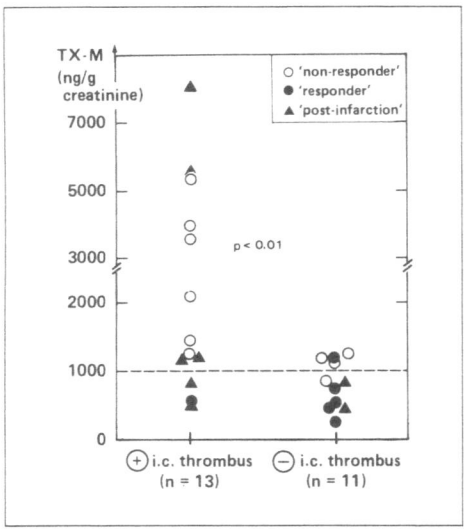

Fig. 2. Excretion of 2,3-dinor-thromboxane B_2 (TX-M) and angiographic evidence of intracoronary (i.c.) thrombus formation in 24 patients with unstable angina. Open circles represent the non-responder group (more than 48-h intravenous nitroglycerine therapy), closed circles represent the responder group, and triangles are the postinfarction patients [7].

The normal range of 2,3-dinor-thromboxane B_2 excretion in this laboratory is 200—1 000 ng/g creatinine; the normal range of 2,3-dinor-6-keto prostaglandin F_1 alpha excretion ranges between 40 and 180 ng/g creatinine.

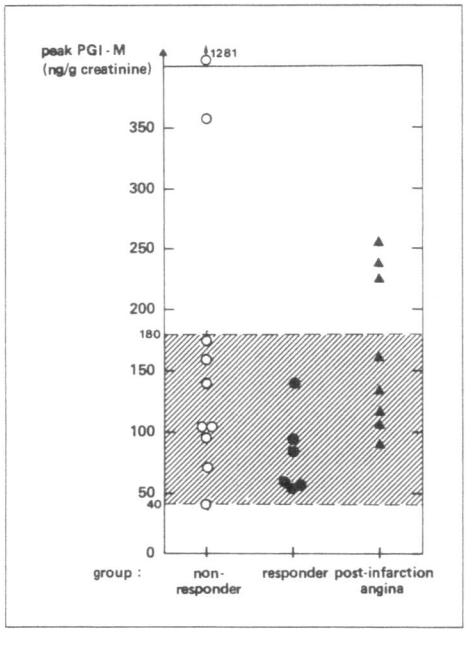

Fig. 3. Urinary excretion of 2,3-dinor-6-keto-prostaglandin F_1alpha (PGI-M) in 24 patients with unstable angina. Only five patients showed evidence of some increase in urinary excretion of PGI-M [7].

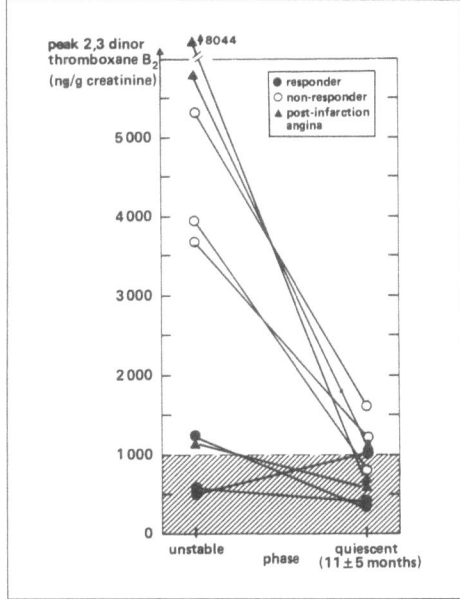

Fig. 4. Urinary excretion of 2,3-dinor-thromboxane B_2 during the acute (unstable) and quiescent phase of nine patients, which were again studied 11 ± 5 months later. Responder and non-responder are classified according to their course during the acute phase [7].

Results

The results are illustrated in Figs. 2—4. Thirteen out of 24 patients showed evidence of an intracoronary thrombus during angiography. All except three patients (two postinfarction and one "responder") showed elevated excretion of thromboxane metabolites during the sampling period. In contrast, those patients without angiographically detectable intracoronary thrombus formation showed normal or only slightly elevated excretion of thromboxane metabolites.

Prostacyclin synthesis was not depressed (Fig. 3), but there was also little evidence, except in two patients of the non responder group, for an elevation of urinary prostacycline metabolites.

All except one of nine patients who underwent follow-up study had undergone coronary artery bypass surgery and were clinically stable. During follow-up (Fig. 4) urine analysis showed values for 2,3-dinor-thromboxane B_2 excretion (854 ± 366 ng/g creatinine) and 2,3-dinor-6-keto prostaglandin F_1alpha (177 ± 151 ng/g creatinine) in the normal or high normal range, irrespective of whether high or low levels were found during the acute, unstable phase.

Fourteen of 24 patients revealed ST segment depression during Holter monitoring; two patients with postinfarction angina showed ST segment elevation. ST segment changes were unrelated to the index of platelet activation.

Discussion

Our results indicate elevated excretion of the major thromboxane A_2 metabolite in patients with unstable angina resistant to medical therapy. They confirm the findings of FitzGerald et al. [6]. Platelet activation, indicated by an elevated excretion of thromboxan A_2 metabolites was not present during follow-up investigation in the quiescent phase.

Furthermore, Vejar et al. [15] recently measured the urinary excretion of 11-dehydro-thromboxane B_2 in patients with unstable angina during treatment with i.v. isosorbiddinitrate and oral diltiazem and found increased levels in nearly half of the patients. 11-dehydro-thromboxane B_2 is the second major metabolite of thromboxan B_2, built by 11-OH-dehydrogenation. Since the physiologic production rate of thromboxane B_2 in the circulation is extremly low, with a maximal estimate of serum thromboxane B_2 concentration in the order of 2 pg/ml, an enhanced excretion rate of TX B_2 metabolites is indicative for platelet activation which occurs episodically in the vast majority of patients.

However, two points should be taken into account:

We cannot rule out that platelets may play only a peripheral or passive role in the pathophysiology of acute coronary syndromes but once activated, may initiate a cycle. One should not interpret the results of platelet activation in unstable angina as a single "cause-effect" relation, because it is difficult to interrupt the pathogenetic sequences by "pure" antiplatelet interventions [10]. Our own data [14] indicate that there is no generalized hypercoagulability of platelets from patients with unstable angina compared to patients with stable, exercise-induced angina. Substances such as adenosin-diphosphate, platelet activating factor, and serotonine released from activated platelets or macrophages may contribute to thrombus formation and vasoreaction as well.

References

1. Bresnahan DR, Davis JL, Holmes DR, Smith HC (1985) Angiographic occurrence and clinical correlates of intraluminal coronary artery thrombus: role of unstable angina. J Am Coll Cardiol 6: 285—289
2. Bugiardini R, Chierchia S, Crea F et al (1984) Evaluation of the effects of catheter sampling for the study of platelet behavior in the pulmonary and coronary circulation. Am Heart J 108: 255—260
3. Capone G, Wolf M, Meyer B, Meister SG (1985) Frequency of intracoronary filling defects by angiography in angina pectoris at rest. Am J Cardiol 56: 403—406
4. Davies MJ, Thomas AC, Knapman OA, Hangartner JR (1986) Intramyocardial platelet aggregation in patients with unstable angina suffering sudden ischemic cardiac death. Circulation 73: 418—427
5. FitzGerald GA, Pedersen AK; Patrono C (1983) Analysis of prostacyclin and thromboxane biosynthesis in cardiovascular disease. Circulation 67: 1174—1177
6. FitzGerald DJ, Roy L, Catella, F, FitzGerald GA (1986) Platelet activation in unstable coronary disease. N Eng J Med 315: 983—989
7. Hamm CW, Lorent, RL, Bleifeld W, Kupper W, Wober W, Weber PC (1987) Biochemical Evidence of platelet activation in patients with persistent unstable angina. J Am Coll Cardiol 10: 998—1004

8. Holmes DR, Hartzler GO, Smith HC, Fuster V (1981) Coronary artery thrombosis in patients with unstable angina. Br Heart J 45: 411—416
9. Nichos AB, Owen J, Grossman BA, Marcella J, Fleisher LN, Lee MML (1984) Effect of heparin bonding on catheter-induced fibrin formation and platelet activation. Circulation 70: 843—850
10. Oates JA, FitzGerald GA, Branch RA, Jackson EK, Knapp HR, Roberts LJ (1988) Clinical implications of prostaglandin and thromboxane A$_2$ formation. N Engl J Med 319: 689—698
11. Patrono C, Ciabattoni G, Pugliese F, Pierucci A, Blair IA, FitzGerald GA (1986) Estimated rate of thromboxane secretion into the circulation of normal humans. J Clin Invest 77: 590—594
12. Roy L, Knapp HR, Robertson RM, Garret A, FitzGerald GA (1985) Endogenous biosynthesis of prostacyclin during cardiac catheterization and angiography in man. Circulation 71: 434—440
13. Sherman TC, Litvack F, Grundfest W (1986) Coronary angioscopy in patients with unstable angina pectoris. N Engl A Med 315: 913—919
14. Terres W, Hamm CW, Kupper W, Bleifeld W (1988) Thrombozytenfunktion bei instabiler Angina pectoris. Dtsch med Wschr 113: 1182—1186
15. Vejar M, Lipkin DP, Maseri A, Bron GVR, Ciabattoni G, Patrono C (1988) Dissociation of platelet activation and spontaneous myocardial ischemia in unstable angina. Clin Res 36: 326A
16. Vetrovec GW, Cowley MJ, Overton H, Richardson DW (1981) Intracoronary thrombus in syndromes of unstable myocardial ischemia. Am Heart J 102: 1202—1208

Authors' address:
W. Kupper, M.D.
Department of Cardiology
Medical Clinic
University Hospital Eppendorf
2000 Hamburg, FRG

Discussion

HUBER:

Do you have data about non-coronary disease with chest pain, for example in patients with a spastic angina or in patients with a psychiatric chest pain syndrome. Do they show also changes in metabolism of prostaglandins?

KUPPER:

No, we have not analyzed this. We have a sample of 150 patients with normal coronary arteries and angina-like chest pain, but we could not do metabolite analyses in these patients.

VON ARNIM:

Would you make a case for the not-so-low dose of aspirin? What is the lowest dose that is sensible and how much do you give regularly?

KUPPER:

The only one reason I can see for a higher dose of aspirin, and I mean 1 500 mg, are the results of Kaltenbach in his PTCA group, who found a significantly reduced re-occlusion rate of 17%. His finding is singular in Europe and the Western Countries, but he has this low restenosis rate and the only difference regarding his patients and the others is the use of this high dose of aspirin, 500 mg three times daily. On the other hand, I think Prof. Patrono has published his results 10 years ago: I agree completely that we come to lower doses of aspirin. What is the effective lowest dose is to my knowledge, addressed in many ongoing clinical trials for between 20 mg and 50 mg. From a theoretical point of view it is clear that there is a complete inhibition of the cyclooxygenase of the platelets with a dose of 20 mg.

PATRONO:

From clinical trials with end points, of prevention of myocardial infarctions, stroke or death, we have no evidence whatsoever that going from 325 up to 1 300 or 1 500 mg makes any difference. That applies also to patients with unstable angina, because the results of the Canadian trial, which uses four-times as much aspirin as the American trial does not show any greater efficacy. If anything, the data from Canada are less convincing. Whether there is any difference between 325 mg and 40 or 50 mg which might be the lowest dose which would fully blank the platelet oxygenase, we do not really know. What I showed today might suggest that low-dose aspirin, even though it causes greater than 95% suppression of platelet cyclo-oxygenase activity, might still leave a small residue amount of enzyme activity which should be sufficient, provided that the stimulus is also very intensive and long-lasting. That is an open question which can only been answered by comparison trials of 40 vs 325 mg.

MASERI:

One problem, that we have discussed more than once, is whether other cells that have the possibility of resynthesizing the enzymes, for example, macrophages in the blood, would be inhibited only for a few hours after the single dose or not. I remember data by Jim Willerson from Dallas, where in cross-sections of the coronary artery in semicircular stenoses show that there is a very intense activity of thromboxane B2 on that side. So it is as if segments of the area which is stenotic and undergoing platelet adhesion in a way picks up the thromboxane as well as serotonin and it is possible that there may be other areas, not necessarily the platelets, that have to be inhibited.

Hemorheologic profile and precursors in myocardial ischemia

M. Leschke and B. E. Strauer

Abteilung für Kardiologie, Pneumologie und Angiologie, Universität Düsseldorf, FRG

Introduction

A discussion of the pathogenesis of unstable angina pectoris involves the consideration of a number of etiological factors that may result in an acute episode of myocardial ischemia. These include critical coronary stenosis [1, 28], coronary arterial spasm due to an increase in vascular tone [25, 31], an increased platelet aggregability [10], coronary thrombosis [17, 24, 42, 45], and increased myocardial oxygen demand during hypertension or tachycardia [31], as well as a decreased synthesis of vasodilatative-acting prostaglandins [38].

An altered blood viscosity as a possible responsible factor in the pathogenesis of angina was initially postulated by Fuchs et al. [8]. Nikolaides et al. [29] discovered that patients with a stable angina showed increased viscosity of whole blood, fibrinogen, and hematocrit levels as well as a decrease in erythrocyte flexibility. A positive correlation between rheological parameters and the severity of coronary artery disease could be demonstrated by Lowe and coworkers [23].

Patients and methods

Unstable angina: In 48 patients that presented at the University Hospital in Marburg, FRG, with symptoms of an unstable angina pectoris between September, 1985 and June, 1986, a detailed rheological diagnostic workup was performed within 24 h of admission. The following criteria were used to define the symptoms based classification of unstable angina.

1) newly arising anginal symptoms of a progressive nature or known anginal symptoms of increasing severity;
2) a lack of significant ST-segment elevation in the extremity or chest leads of the ECG;
3) persistence of anginal symptoms under a maximal orally administered antianginal medication of nitrates, β-blockers, and calcium antagonists;
4) no elevation of serum creatine kinase levels above 120 U/l (normal value less than 80 U/l).

In all patients fulfilling the above mentioned criteria, and thus diagnosed as having unstable angina, a coronary angiography was performed within four days after admission.

Stable angina: 83 patients with stable anginal symptoms and angiographically documented coronary artery disease presenting at the University Hospital in the above mentioned time span, were also examined for parameters of blood rheology.

Myocardial infarction: 45 patients suffering from acute myocardial infarction were also examined for parameters of blood rheology within 24 h of initial symptoms. At the time of blood withdrawal the patients had received no thrombolytic therapy. The treatment involved intravenous application of heparin (1 000—1 500 IU/h) and sodiumdinitrate (trinitrosan, 1—6 mg/h) as well as nifedipin (n = 8) (adalat 0.6—1.2 mg/h).

Control group: 34 normotensive patients with no angiographic indication of coronary artery disease and cardiomyopathy represented the control group.

Rheological analysis: 20 ml of venous blood anticoagulated with EDTA were drawn from each patient. Hematocrit, plasma viscosity, erythrocyte aggregation rate and whole blood viscosity were determined from the sample. To determine the plasma fibrinogen levels using the Ouchterlony technique (Partigenplates Behringwerke) 5 ml of blood was made uncoaguable with sodium citrate. Hematocrit, plasma viscosity, and whole blood viscosity were determined at 37 °C on the OCRD measuring device (Fa. Anton Paar, Graz, Austria) according to Chmiel [5]. The erythrocyte aggregation rates were measured in the erythrocyte aggregometer MA-1 (Fa. Myrenne, Roetgen, Germany) according to H. Schmid-Schönbein [35] at a hematocrit of 0.35.

The relative viscosity determined as the quotient of whole blood viscosity (at a shear rate of $\gamma = 2/s$ and a hematocrit of 0.35), and plasma viscosity serve to characterize the intrinsic rheological properties of erythrocytes, independent of plasma viscosity, as well as erythrocyte aggregation and hematocrit.

Whole blood count, serum cholesterol and serum triglycerides were determined in all patients. With respect to the patient's history patients' reports of cigarette smoking were recorded. Blood pressure was measured on the reclining patient using a blood pressure cuff according to Riva-Rocci.

Coronary angiography: the coronary angiography involved a flotation catheter, coronary angiography, and a monoplanar ventriculography in 30 ° RAO. The cardiac index was determined via thermodilution, the left ventricular ejection fraction (EF) ventriculographically was determined with the help of a computer-assisted quantification technique. The severity of the coronary artery disease was classified as a I, II or III vessel disease (significant stenosis more than 50 %) and a coronary score was established in accordance with American Heart Association criteria [3]. Severe stenosis over 90 % were listed separately.

Statistics: the rheological and clinico-chemical parameters were documented as means ± standard deviations. If the data from the various groups differed significantly in an analysis of variance [4], an additional statistical workup using Student's *t*-test for two-dimensional variance was performed. Differences were considered statistically significant at a probability of error of 5 %.

Results

Clinical (Table 1) and laboratory data (Table 2): the examined population, mainly men, was of comparable age. Two-thirds of those with coronary artery disease were

Table 1: Clinical data.

	Controls	Stable Angina pectoris	Unstable Angina pectoris	Myocardial Infarction
age	55 ± 10	60 ± 8	60 ± 9	68 ± 12*
sex	23♂, 11♀	68♂, 15♀	41♂, 7♀	30♂, 15♀
smoker	9	18	20	16
		66%	68%	58%
exsmoker	?	37	12	10
non-smoker	25	28	16	19
medication				
nitrates	20	32	28	26
betablocker	1	21	12	11
Ca-channel-blocker	3	39	30	28

* $p < 0.01$

Table 2: Laboratory data.

	Controls	Stable Angina	Unstable Angina	Myocardial Infarction
Leukocytes [μl']	6100 ± 1700	6900 ± 1600	8400 ± 2600**[1,2]	10600 ± 2600**[1,2,3]
Platelets [10^3 μl']	268 ± 73*[4]	229 ± 67	245 ± 59*[4]	209 ± 58
Triglycerides [mg/dl]	150 ± 70	209 ± 39*[1,4]	222 ± 182*[1,4]	141 ± 58
Cholesterol [mg/dl]	223 ± 60	237 ± 47	240 ± 57	230 ± 57
Creatine phosphokinase [U/l]	–	48 ± 29 (n = 56)	59 ± 29 (n = 48)	519 ± 418**[2,3]

* $p < 0.01$, ** $p < 0.001$
[1] vs controls, [2] vs stable AP, [3] vs unstable AP, [4] vs AMI

smokers or exsmokers. Those suffering from myocardial infarction showed higher diastolic blood pressures. No differences were seen in the antianginous therapy used before hospital admission in the three groups suffering from coronary artery disease. Thus potential effects of the medication used toward the parameters of blood rheology results could be ignored.

The highest white blood cell count (wcc) was determined in those patients suffering from myocardial infarction; patients with unstable angina had counts higher than those with stable angina. Lowest wcc was found in patients with normal coronary arteries. The blood platelet count was decreased in patients suffering from myocardial infarction. With the exception of a lower level of triglycerides in the myocardial infarction patients serum lipid levels showed no significant differences among the three groups with coronary artery disease. Creatine kinase levels were slightly but not significantly higher in patients with unstable angina than in those with stable angina.

Table 3: Hemodynamic and coronary angiography results.

	Stable Angina	Unstable Angina
systolic RR	146 ± 25	143 ± 30
diastolic RR [mmHg]	83 ± 12	78 ± 15
cardiac Index [l/min · m²]	3.5 ± 0.9 (n = 72)	3.1 ± 0.7 (n = 47)
ejection fraction [%]	58.2 ± 16.5 (n = 56)	61.5 ± 14.3 (n = 34)
I -vessel-CAD	15	17
II -vessel-CAD	25	8
III -vessel-CAD	43	23
No. of patients with stenosis ≥ 90%	61 (73%)	43 (89%)
No. of stenosis ≥ 90% per patient	1.7 ± 1.4	1.8 ± 1.6
mean coronary score	12.3 ± 6.4	13.7 ± 5.6

Hemodynamic and coronary angiography results (Table 3): Cardiac index and ejection fraction showed no significant difference between patients with stable and unstable angina. Fifty percent of the patients with stable or unstable angina showed a three-vessel disease. Patients with unstable angina frequently revealed single-vessel disease. The extent of higher degrees of stenosis (greater than 90 %) was distinctly higher in patients with unstable angina (89 %) than in those with stable anginal symptoms (73 %). The frequency of high-degree coronary stenosis and the mean coronary score were slightly but not significantly increased in patients with unstable angina.

Blood rheology (Tables 4 and 5): Plasma fibrinogen, plasma viscosity, and erythrocyte aggregation rate were found to be comparable in patients with unstable angina and myocardial infarction, however, they were significantly higher than in patients presenting with stable angina. In comparison to the control group patients with stable angina revealed somewhat higher levels in all parameters.

In this analysis whole blood viscosity as an unspecific global parameter of rheology was only taken into account at a shear rate of $\gamma = 2s^{-1}$. The slight increase in whole blood viscosity in unstable angina and myocardial infarction can be explained by the increase in plasma viscosity and erythrocyte aggregation rate, which together with the hematocrit and erythrocyte deformability determine whole blood viscosity. Due to a high degree of variance whole blood viscosity does not distinguish between patients with a normal coronary angiogram and patients with stable angina. The elevated relative viscosity values obtained from patients with unstable angina and myocardial infarction suggest the presence of rigid erythrocytes.

Table 4: Rheological data.

	Controls	Stable Angina	Unstable Angina	Myocardial Infarction
Fibrinogen [mg/dl]	227.3 ± 50.4 (n = 16)	295.3 ± 68.6*[1] (n = 44)	394.4 ± 82.7*[1,2] (n = 33)	390.2 ± 126.9*[1,2] (n = 27)
Plasma Viscosity [mPas]	1.24 + 0.07 (n = 34)	1.33 ± 0.08**[1] (n = 78)	1.39 ± 0.08**[1,2] (n = 48)	1.37 ± 0.09**[1,2] (n = 45)
RBC Aggregation [hct 0.35]	9.6 ± 3.2 (n = 28)	13.1 ± 3.1**[1] (n = 42)	15.8 ± 3.2**[1,2] (n = 46)	14.7 ± 4.3*[1,2] (n = 37)
Hematocrit	0.43 ± 0.03 (n = 31)	0.43 ± 0.05 (n = 80)	0.43 ± 0.03 (n = 46)	0.43 ± 0.04 (n = 43)
Whole Blood Viscosity [mPas]	6.79 ± 1.02 (n = 32)	7.32 ± 0.96 (n = 76)	7.71 ± 1.02*[1,2] (n = 45)	7.62 ± 1.42 (n = 40)
Relative Viscosity	3.92 ± 0.27 (n = 31)	3.88 ± 0.27 (n = 72)	4.02 ± 0.25**[2] (n = 42)	3.95 ± 0.27 (n = 39)

* $p < 0.02$, ** $p < 0.01$; 1. vs. controls, 2. vs. stable angina.

Table 5: Plasma viscosity [mPas] related to severity of CAD.

	Stable Angina	Unstable Angina
I -vessel-CAD	1.27 ± 0.07 (n = 15)	1.36 ± 0.04** (n = 17)
II -vessel-CAD	1.31 ± 0.08 (n = 25)	1.36 ± 0.06 (n = 8)
III -vessel-CAD	1.34 ± 0.09 (n = 43)	1.41 ± 0.07* (n = 23)

* $p < 0.01$, ** $p < 0.001$.

Table 5 shows the plasma viscosity in patients with stable and unstable angina classified according to degree of coronary vessel disease. Within the patients groups showing stable or unstable angina, patients with coronary three-vessel disease presented higher plasma viscosity than those with single-vessel disease. In patients with comparable coronary angiographic findings those suffering from unstable angina revealed higher plasma viscosity levels than those with stable symptoms.

Discussion

According to our results plasma viscosity and plasma fibrinogen levels are raised in unstable angina in contrast to stable angina, whereby the rheological changes increase with the severity of coronary artery disease.

From a rheological point of view it is furthermore important to note that plasma viscosity as the decisive rheological determinant of microcirculation shows an increase before the manifestation of overt myocardial infarction. These changes are thus not to be interpreted as secondary occurrences but rather more as a significant factor in the pathogenesis of progression of unstable angina to myocardial ischemia and coronary thrombogenesis.

The pathologically raised plasma viscosity is a consequence of the hyperfibrinogenemia. The fibrinogen molecule as macromolecule (rel. molecular mass 341, 000) and determinant of plasma viscosity must thus be considered to take a central position in the rheological changes occurring in coronary artery disease. Apparently, unstable angina is characterized by a rise in plasma fibrinogen analogous to an "acute phase reaction," showing a steady progression toward myocardial infarction.

As a number of authors have reported [6, 11], myocardial infarction presents with a further rise in plasma fibrinogen levels, plasma viscosity, and erythrocyte aggregation; these may depend on the infarct size and degree of an infarct-induced inflammatory reaction.

Which mechanism is finally responsible for the initial increase in plasma fibrinogen levels in unstable angina is, as of yet, not known. Elevated plasma fibrinogen levels measured in patients with degenerative vascular diseases [2] are also found in stable angina. It is possible that these increased fibrinogen levels in degenerative vascular disease are the consequence of a chronic increase in fibrinogen turnover in atherosclerotic lesions [12, 39, 41]. On the other hand, relationships have been shown between plasma fibrinogen and the extent of coronary artery disease [20], and cardiovascular risk factors such as hyperlipidemia [19, 37, 40], hypertension [22], and cigarette smoking [18, 40]. An etiological link between cardiovascular risk factors and hyperfibrinogenemia has not yet determined. According to new research within the scope of the "Framingham Study" [13, 14], the "Northwick-Park Heart Study" [27], as well as results from Wilhelmsen and colleagues [43] shows that plasma fibrinogen is being considered as an independent cardiovascular risk factor in its own right in the pathogenesis of coronary artery disease.

It cannot be ruled out that the slightly higher proportion of critical degrees of coronary stenosis in patients presenting with unstable angina is significant for the hyperfibrinogenemia. To what extent endothelial lesions and ruptures in the vascular intima at sites of critical coronary stenosis can initiate local ischemia and thereby induce inflammatory reactions involving mediation by prostaglandins, granulocytes, and macrophages, remains unclear. According to kinetic studies making use of radioactively marked fibrinogen and following an appropriate stimulus, fibrinogen levels are shown to rise within 2 h due to induction of hepatic synthesis [41]. In conjunction with these findings concerning the significance of inflammatory processes in the pathogenesis of unstable angina, a study [15] is of interest in which during autopsy of 12 patients whose deaths were related to unstable angina, focal inflammatory infiltrates within the adventitia were documented. Furthermore, it is possible to interpret the findings of raised white blood cell counts in patients with stable angina and coronary arery disease [16] as a "chronic inflammatory reaction" within the coronary vessels. The elevated white blood cell count of patients with unstable angina may lead to an interference in the microcirculation of the ischemic myocardium [7, 33] due to the rather large cell diameter of polymorphonuclear neutrophils in respect to the capillary diameter and due to the almost 1 000-fold higher membrane rigidity in comparison to erythrocytes [33].

90

In a modern analysis of the pathogenetic significance of parameters of blood rheology on unstable angina one must make use of theoretical considerations and experimental results of normal and abnormal hemorheology, as well as the most recent clinical data. The normally high degree of blood fluidity in areas of low shear stresses in the microvasculature is decreased due to an increase in plasma viscosity, in erythrocytes aggregation and rigidity, in white blood cell activation, and as a consequence of an exhaustion of vasomotor capacity, in poststenotic vascular segments [34]. This reduction in blood fluidity and consecutive increase in viscous resistance further supports another experimentally identified mechanism, the "collateral viscidification" [36], which in turn leads to a further reduction in collateral capillary flow encouraging ischemia. According to theoretical calculations [9] an increase in blood viscosity already involves the reduction of the peripheral oxygen release. Indirect evidence can be deducted from results of a fibrinogen- and viscosity-lowering therapy with low dose urokinase in patients with therapy-resistant angina [21]; in these patients a decreased frequency of angina and increased tolerance of physical strain could be noted due to fibrinogenolysis and thereby, improved myocardial perfusion. Findings of elevated plasma fibrinogen levels as well as an altered plasma viscosity and a reduction in fibrinolytic potential in coronary artery disease led to the concept of hypercoagulability [26, 30, 44], as a significant factor in the increased thrombogenic tendency and in the progression of coronary artery disease. The pathogenic mechanism by which an increase in whole blood viscosity influences myocardial ischemia is shown in Fig. 1.

In conclusion, it is possible to propose that patients suffering from coronary artery disease with stable angina differ from "healthy patients" in that they show a chronic hyperfibrinogenemia equivalent to an inflammatory reaction of the vascular bed.

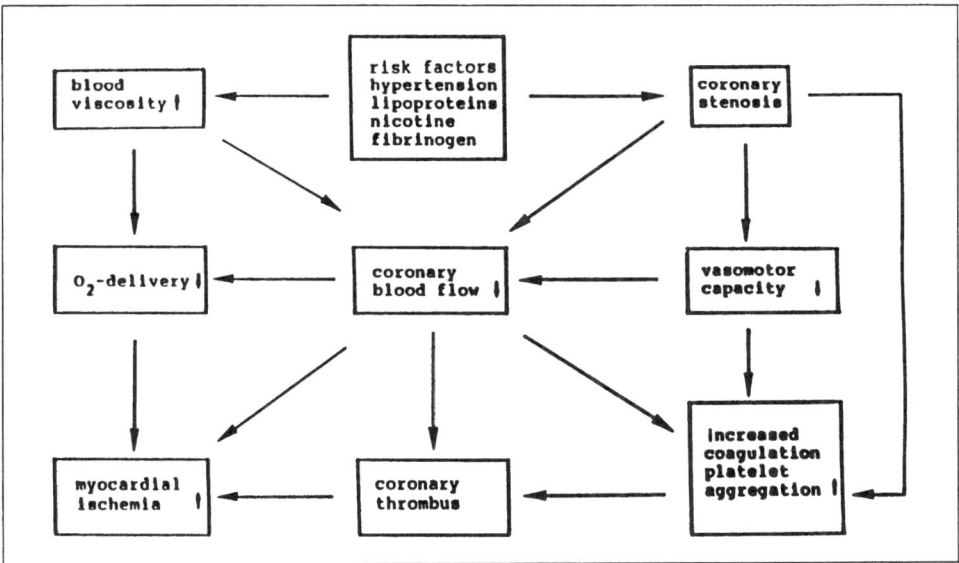

Fig. 1. Blood viscosity and myocardial ischemia.

In unstable angina an acute phase reaction with an additional increase of fibrinogen occurring before the manifestation of overt myocardial infarction is in part responsible for the clinical instability and preinfarct stage. Thus increase in plasma viscosity and fibrinogen may contribute to the progression of ischemia and its clinical sequel of symptoms in unstable angina pectoris.

References

1. Ambrose JA, Winters SL, Stern A, Eng A, Teichholz LE, Gorlin R, Fuster V (1985) Angiographic morphology and the pathogenesis of unstable angina pectoris. J Am Coll Cardiol 5: 609
2. Angelkort B, Gerlach A, Schabner W, Mäder A, Spürk P (1984) Blutfluidität bei chronischer peripherer Verschlußkrankheit. In: Heilmann L, Kiesewetter H, Ernst E (eds) Klinische Rheologie und Beta-1-Blockade. Zuckerschwerdt, München—Bern—Wien, p 58
3. Austen WG, Edwards JE, Frye RL, Gensini GG, Gott VL, Griffith LSC, McGoon DC, Murphy ML, Roe BB (1976) A reporting system on patients evaluated for coronary artery disease. Report of the Ad Hoc Committee for Grading of Coronary Artery Disease. Council on Cardiovascular Surgery, American Heart Association. Circulation 51: 5
4. Bortz J (1985) Lehrbuch der Statistik. 2. Aufl. Springer, Berlin—Heidelberg—New York
5. Chmiel H (1979) Determination of blood rheological parameters and clinical application. Adv Cardiovasc Physiol 3: 1
6. Dodds AJ, Boyd MJ, Allen J, Bennett ED, Flute PT, Dormandy JA (1980) Changes in red cell deformability and other hemorheological variables after myocardial infarction. Brit Heart J 44: 508
7. Engler RL, Dahlgren MD, Morris DD, Petersen MA, Schmid-Schönbein GW (1986) Role of leukocytes in response to acute myocardial ischemia and reflow in dogs. Am J Physiol 241: H314
8. Fuchs J, Weinberger I, Rotenberger Z, Erdberg A, Davidson E, Joshna H, Agmon J (1984) Plasma viscosity in ischemic heart disease. Am Heart J 108: 435
9. Gordon RJ, Snyder GK, Titel H, Taylor WJ (1975) Potential significance of plasma viscosity and hematocrit variations in myocardial infarction. Circulation 51: 1079
10. Hirsh PD, Hillis LD, Campbell WB, Firth BG, Willerson JT (1981) Release of prostaglandins and thromboxane into the coronary circulation in patients with ischemic heart disease. New Engl J Med 304: 685
11. Jan KM, Chien S, Bigger JT (1975) Observations on blood viscosity changes after acute myocardial infarction. Circulation 51: 1079
12. Kadish JL (1979) Fibrin and atherogenesis — a hypothesis. Atherosclerosis 33: 409
13. Kannel WB (1987) Fibrinogen, cigarette smoking, and risk of cadiovascular disease. Insights from the Framingham Study. J Am Coll Cardiol 9: 78A
14. Kannel WB, Wolf PA, Castelli WP, D'Agostino RB (1987) Fibrinogen and risk of cardiovascular disease. J Am Med Assoc 258: 1183
15. Kohchi K, Takebayaski S, Tadayuki H, Nobuyoski M (1985) Significance of adventitial inflammation of the coronary artery in patients with unstable angina: results at autopsy. Circulation 71: 709
16. Kostis JB, Turkevich D, Sharp J (1984) Association between leukocyte count and the presence and extent of coronary atherosclerosis as determined by coronary angiography. Am J Cardiol 53: 997
17. Krushal JB, Commerford PJ, Franks JJ, Kirsch RE (1987) Fibrin and fibrinogen-related antigens in patients with stable and unstable coronary artery disease. New Eng J Med 317: 1361
18. Leonhardt H, Uthoff A, Uthoff C (1977) Vollblut- und Plasmaviskosität bei koronaren Risikofaktoren. Klin Wschr 55: 481
19. Leonhardt H, Arntz HR, Klemens UH (1977) Studies of plasma viscosity in primary hyperlipoproteinaemia. Atherosclerosis 28: 29
20. Leschke M, Motz W, Strauer BE (1986) Hämorheologisch-therapeutische Anwendungsmöglichkeiten bei der koronaren Herzerkrankung. Münch Med Wochenschr 136: 17S
21. Leschke M, Blanke H, Motz W, Höffken H, Strauer BE (1987) Low dose urokinase treatment in patients with therapy refractory angina pectoris. Clin Hemorheol 7: 401

22. Letcher RL, Chien S, Pickering TG, Laragh JH (1983) Elevated blood viscosity in patients with borderline essential hypertension. Hypertension 5: 757
23. Lowe GDO, Drummond MM, Lorimer AR, Hutton I, Forbes CD, Prentice CRM, Barbenel JC (1980) Relation between extent of coronary artery disease and blood viscosity. Brit Med J: 673
24. Mandelkorn JB, Nelson MW, Singh S, Shechter JA, Kersh RI, David MR, Workman MB, Bentivoglio LG, LaPorte SM, Meister SG (1983) Intracoronary thrombus in nontransmural myocardial infarction and in unstable angina pectoris. Am J Cardiol 52: 1
25. Maseri A (1981) The revival of coronary spasm. Am J Med 70: 752
26. Meade TW, Chakrabarti R, Haines AP, North WRS, Stirling Y (1979) Characteristics affecting fibrinolytic activity and plasma fibrinogen concentration. Br Med J: 153
27. Meade TW, Chakrabarti R, Haines AP, North WRS, Stirling Y, Thompson SG (1980) Haemostatic function and cardiovascular death: early results of a prospective study. Lancet 17: 1050
28. Moise A, Theroux P, Taeymanns Y, Descoings B, Lesperance J, Waters DD, Pelletier GB, Bourassa MG (1983) Unstable angina and progression of coronary atherosclerosis. N Eng J Med 309: 685
29. Nicolaides AN, Horbourne T, Boneers R, Kidner PH, Besterman EM (1977) Blood viscosity, red-cell flexibility, haematocrit and plasma-fibrinogen in patients with angina. Lancet 5: 943
30. O'Connor NTY, Cederholm-Williams S, Copper S, Cotter L (1984) Hypercoagulability and coronary artery disease. Br Heart J 52: 614
31. Rafflenbeul W, Lichtlen PR (1982) The concept of "dynamic" coronary artery stenosis. Z Kardiol 71: 439
32. Roughgarden JW (1966) Circulatory changes associated with spontaneous angina pectoris. Am J Med 41: 947
33. Schmid-Schönbein GW, Engler RL (1986) Granulocytes as active participants in acute myocardial ischemia and infarction. Am J Cardiovasc Pathol 1: 15
34. Schmid-Schönbein H (1981) Myokardiale Mikrozirkulation: Wechselwirkung zwischen Vasomotorik und Fließeigenschaften des Blutes. Dt Med Wschr 106: 1483
35. Schmid-Schönbein H, Volger E, Teitel P, Kiesewetter H, Dauer U, Heilmann L (1982) New hemorheological techniques for the routine laboratory. Clin Hemorheology 2: 93
36. Schmid-Schönbein H (1982) Physiologie und Pathologie der Mikrozirkulation aus rheologischer Sicht. Internist 23: 359
37. Seplowitz AH, Chien S, Smith FR (1981) Effects of lipoproteins of plasma viscosity. Atherosclerosis 38: 89
38. Serneri GGN, Gensini GF, Abbate R, Prisco D, Rogasi PG, Laurano R, Casalo GC, Fautini F, Di Donato M, Dabizzi RP (1985) Abnormal cardiocoronary thromboxane A2 production in patients with unstable angina. Am Heart J 109: 732
39. Smith EB, Smith RH (1976) Early changes in aortic intima. Atherosclerosis Rev 1: 119
40. Stoltz JF (1981) Cardiovascular disease, risk factors and hemorheological parameters. Clin Hemorheology 3: 257
41. Stuart J (1984) the acute phase reaction and haematological stress syndrome in vascular disease. Int J Microcirc: Clin Exp 3: 11
42. Vetrovec GW, Cowley MJ, Overton H, Richardson DW (1981) Intracoronary thrombus in syndromes of unstable myocardial ischemia. Am Heart J 102: 1202
43. Wilhelmsen L, Svärdsudd K, Korsan-Bengtsen K, Larsson B, Welin L, Tibblin G (1984) Fibrinogen as a risk factor for stroke and myocardial infarction. N Engl J Med 311: 501
44. Yornell JWG, Sweetnam PM, Elwood PC, Eastham R, Gilmour RA, O'Brian JR, Etherington MD (1985) Haemostatic factors and ischaemic heart disease. The Caerphilly Study. Br Heart J 53: 483
45. Zack PM, Ischinger T, Akter UT, Dincer B, Kennedy HL (1984) The occurrence of angiographically detected intracoronary thrombus in patients with unstable angina pectoris. Am Heart J 1984: 1408

Authors' address:
Dr. Matthias Leschke
Medizinische Einrichtungen der Universität Düsseldorf
Abteilung für Kardiologie, Pneumologie und Angiologie
Moorenstraße 5
D-4000 Düsseldorf 1, FRG

Discussion

KRUCOFF:

How many of the processes you describe might be exacerbated by the chronic dehydration that a good number of patients with acute myocardial infarction or unstable syndromes present with. Is just a lack of serum water a potential contributor?

LESCHKE:

I would not say that dehydration plays any significant role in this mechanism. It is however described in patients with acute myocardial infarction.

VON ARNIM:

This could be answered by another very important parameter for viscosity, which I wonder why you did not include. That is the hematocrit. In all studies on parameters of viscosity the hematocrit seems to be very important. Why did you leave it out?

LESCHKE:

We could not find any differences in these patients groups in respect to the hematocrit values. We think that whole-blood viscosity and hematocrit are factors of the macrovessels, but the rheological properties in the microvessels are mostly influenced by plasma viscosity, red-blood-cell aggregation, and fibrinogen. The hematocrit values in the microvessels are about 15—20 %, admost independent of the hematocrit measured.

KRUCOFF:

Another factor in the microvasculature that has been attended to in different settings is red-blood-cell deformability. Did you have the opportunity to examine that in these different groups?

LESCHKE:

We had the opportunity to measure red-blood-cell deformability, and I measured it for about one-and-a-half years in the laboratory. I nearly gave it up because I think it is a rather weak factor in the clinical situation. We did not detect any differences of red-blood-cell deformability in these patients.

DE CATERINA:

In order to distinguish between elevations of fibrinogen due to acute-phase reactions and primary elevations of fibrinogen, would it be easy to measure other indexes of inflammation like c-reactive protein or erythrocyte sedimentation rate in these patients?

LESCHKE:

We tried to measure other factors of the acute-phase reaction, but we could not detect any differences of CRP.

LEMMER:

Since we discussed circadian rhythms this morning, I want to remind you that in 1974, Ailey and coworkers published on circadian variations in hematocrit as well as blood viscosity, with peak values in the early morning, which nicely coincides with the peak value in myocardial infarction.

LESCHKE:

I know the data of Ailey. But there was no relation of time to the parameters of viscosity in our patients. It may well be that the results are influenced by the circadian rhythm.

CHIERCHIA:

You presented the group data and you correlated those group data with the anatomic severity of coronary artery disease. Did you try to correlate the data in terms of fibrinogen and blood viscosity, in general, with the clinical state of the patients? In other words, with disease activity rather than the degree of anatomical damage? If so, was there a stronger correlation?

LESCHKE:

Well, there is a relation between the severity of coronary artery disease and rheological parameters. On the other hand, there is also a correlation to the clinical state. Patients with unstable angina had higher viscosity levels already early on.

ANDREOTTI:

On reason why the CRP may not have correlated with fibrinogen is that it is a slow-reacting acute phase reactant. It takes about five days to reach its peak following myocardial infarction, for instance. I also have a question. Were you able to match your different groups for age and smoking habits, since these two parameters are related with increasing levels of fibrinogen in plasma?

LESCHKE:

The patients were matched in respect to smoking habits, and in every group there were about two-thirds smokers and ex-smokers. And they did not influence the fibrinogen levels. Ex-smokers and smokers have a tendency to higher fibrinogen levels — but in a much greater population, not in these groups of patients. The patient groups were rather similar in their age contribution: 58 years was the mean age, the control group was younger.

HUBER:

Which of your parameters do you think is the most important parameter in coming to myocardial ischemia? Do you think it's fibrinogen?

LESCHKE:

I think that fibrinogen is a very important parameter. On the other hand, the plasma viscosity is a global parameter to describe changes in lipoprotein profile in coagulation, and it is a more global parameter. I would take both parameters into account.

Electrocardiographic patterns of impending coronary closure independent of unstable anginal symptoms

M. W. Krucoff, Y. R. Jackson, K. S. Stark*, K. M. Kent*

Duke University Medical Center, Durham, North Carolina
*Georgetown University Hospital, Washington, D.C., USA

Nonsurgical revascularization with thrombolytic agents or angioplasty (PTCA) technique creates, as a part of the therapeutic effect, an unstable coronary site. Thrombolytic agents dissolve the platelet/thrombin clot, but may not alter the underlying ruptured plaque that first stimulated the thrombogenic cascade. PTCA balloon inflations fracture and tear plaque-imbedded coronary intima, creating a nidus of inflammation and fresh collagen exposure.

Angiographic assessment is most commonly used to assess the success or failure of an intracoronary interevention with thrombolytic agents or PTCA. This primarily anatomic parameter, however, is not always reliable, and 2—30 % of "successfully" dilated or reperfused patients will silently or symptomatically reocclude their intervention site while recuperating in the coronary care unit (CCU) [1—11]. Thus, in the course of their therapy, these patients provide a unique opportunity to study the transition of a coronary nidus from a relatively stable to an unstable state. In addition, patient-specific, coronary site specific data may be gathered for each of these patients during their reference event, either during the MI at presentation or during transient coronary occlusion at PTCA. This reference event may provide additional insight into the patterns seen with recurrent instability.

Continuous multi-lead electrocardiographic surveillance follows ST segment changes as a noninvasive physiologic marker of transient or persistent myocardial ischemia. While less sensitive or specific than other more cumbersome or invasive techniques, ST segment monitoring devices have developed a remarkable new potential for research and clinical applications with the integration of microprocessor technology, allowing multi-lead signal processing and algorithmic/artificial intelligence programming to function in real time at the bedside.

Continuous ST segment monitoring using retrospective 1- or 2-channel devices has been applied to measure or justify medical therapy in chronic situations even in the absence of patient symptoms [12—17]. Continuous ST monitoring has also been shown to be a sensitive and specific noninvasive marker of changes in coronary patency [18, 19]. In most patients, sudden occlusion of a coronary site can be detected in 10—40 s, if the appropriate surface ECG leads are monitored [20—22]. In patients in the CCU following intracoronary interventions, the ability to detect an unstable coronary site prior to patient awareness could allow much earlier medical or invasive therapy, with the potential to markedly reduce the extent of or even prevent myocardial necrosis. Application of such therapies in asymptomatic patients, however, takes on greater significance due to the attendant risks of the therapies themselves.

We have explored the natural history of ST segment changes after intracoronary interventions using newly available digital, microprocessor-based multi-lead ST devices in an effort to better define patterns that identify impending or actual reclosure of a coronary intervention site independent of patient symptoms. This report is an update of previous work with elective PTCA [22, 23] with the addition of a preliminary look at patients receiving thrombolytic therapy and/or emergency PTCA for acute MI.

Methods

A total of 10 375 h of continuous ST segment monitoring was performed during and after 2463 angiographically documented coronary occlusions (acute MI or elective PTCA) in 524 consecutive patients felt to have had a successful intracoronary intervention at the Georgetown University Medical Center. "Success" was defined in all cases based on angiographic criteria. All clinical decisions on subsequent patient management were made in the fashion standard for the Medical Center. Routine CPK's, arrhythmia monitoring, and close clinical attention by bedside nursing staff constituted the standard CCU surveillance. Clinical endpoints assessed in our observations were: MI, urgent bypass surgery, sudden death or death after elective PTCA and MI extension, urgent bypass surgery, sudden death or death after thrombolytic therapy or emergency PTCA.

In the initial phase of our experience, a three-channel Holter monitor (Scole Alta-II) was paired with a fully digitizing playback scanner (Marquette 8000) to give high resolution (mean ST level every 10—15 s) ST analysis on normally conducted beats in three bipolar vectors. This system has been previously described in detail [24]. An example of the output of this system in seen in Figs. 1 and 2.

In the latter phase of this effort, a 12-lead real-time portable programmable microprocessor-driven ST electrocardiograph (Mortara ELI-ST) was evolved and applied. This system acquires a standard 12-lead ECG simultaneously in 12 leads, digitizing the analogue waveforms in real time and comparing them to the patient's own baseline every 30 s. Further retrospective analysis of the digital information can also be performed using graphic and superimposition software developed on an IBM-PC (Interventional Cardiology Associates); this system has been described in a previous publication [25]. Examples of the output of this system are seen in Fgs. 3 and 4.

ST segment fingerprint

We have previously described the temporal stability of patient-specific coronary site-specific multi-lead precordial patterns of ST deviation, or ST "fingerprints" [24]. Despite marked differences in amplitude of ST deviation, recurrent coronary occlusion reproduced the precordial ST fingerprint seen with initial coronary occlusion in 80—90 % of patients over as long as a one-month period in an "all comers" pop-

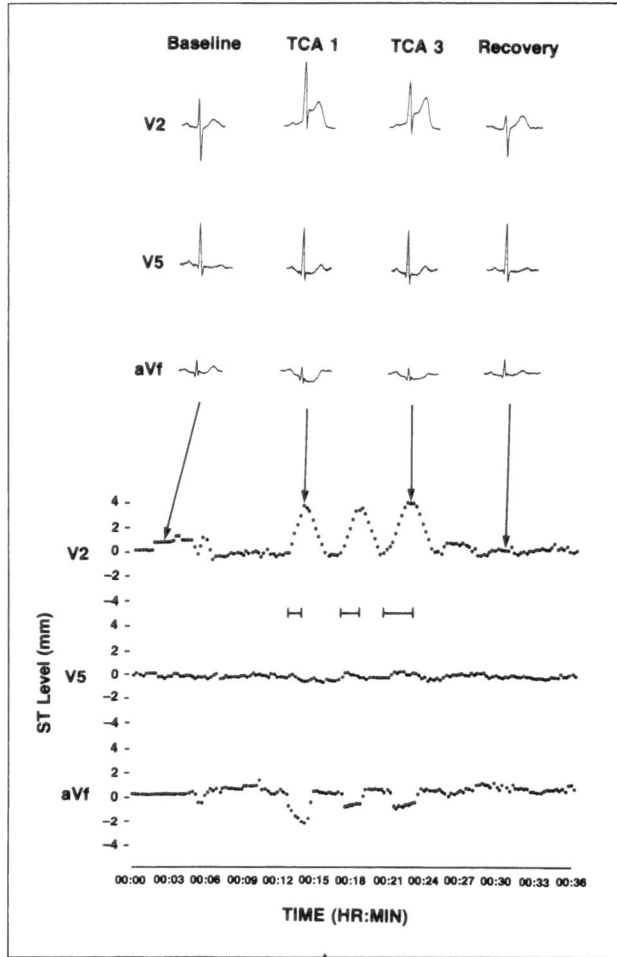

Fig. 1. High resolution ST segment trend from three-channel Holter record/playback. PTCA ballon inflations are indicated by horizontal bars. Trend dots represent mean ST level of normally conducted beats in 15-s periods. Anterior (V2) injury current during each inflation detects and characterizes transient coronary occlusions; inferior (aVf) ST depression detects transient ischemia but does not characterize total occlusion; inferolateral (V5) lead shows less than 1 mm ST deviation, completely missing transient ischemia. Pattern is reproduced over all three leads with each repeat inflation. (Reprinted with permission from [22].)

ulation with reocclusions either during PTCA, in the CCU following PTCA, or with repeat PTCA for restenosis. Identical or clearly related vs different patterns in comparing transient episodes to reference events are determined on the basis of the center of injury current over the precordium, as has been detailed [24].

Results

Temporal stability of the fingerprint pattern, while a necessary condition for application of a monitoring strategy aimed at identifying high risk patients who merit aggressive therapy, does not prove the clinical significance or usefulness of such a strategy per se. Our hypothesis was that the mere detection of ST deviation or no ST deviation might identify statistically different prognostic subgroups, but not with

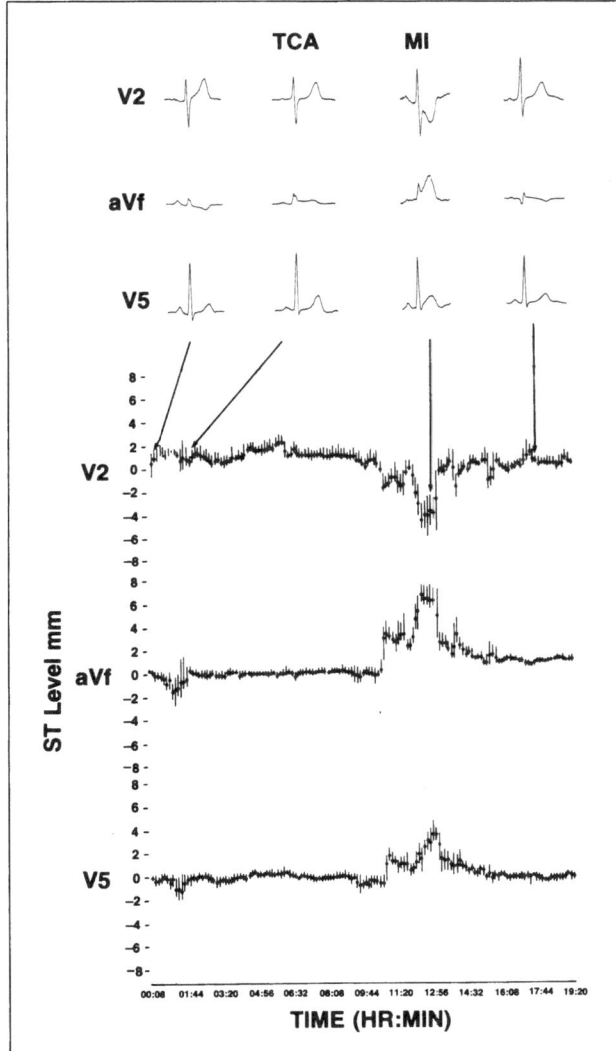

Fig. 2. Low resolution ST segment trend from three-channel Holter. Vertical marks show the range and horizontal marks the mean ST level of normal beats in every 10 min of recording. Inferolateral ST elevation and reciprocal anterior ST depression seen during angioplasty (TCA) is reproduced in greater magnitude during spontaneous closure and acute MI 9 h later in CCU. Patient was completely asymptomatic during MI (Reprinted with permission from [22]).

sufficient specificity to be useful in considering risk-laden therapies in asymptomatic patients. We hypothesized that additional qualitative information with independent prognostic importance, such as the presence or absence of ST segment elevation, and the use of patient-specific, coronary-specific information obtainable in these patients from the reference intracoronary intervention event, might help refine specificity without a significant loss in sensitivity in the identification of high risk patients.

Retrospective review of the occurrence of clinical endpoints across our patient population based on the presence or absence of ST deviation, based on the presence or absence of ST elevation, and based on the presence or absence of ST elevation

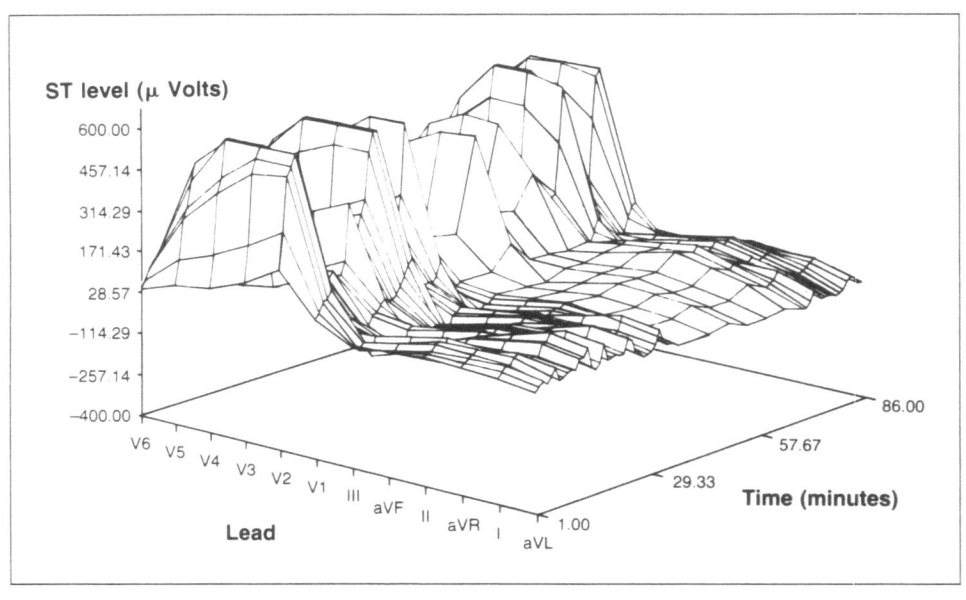

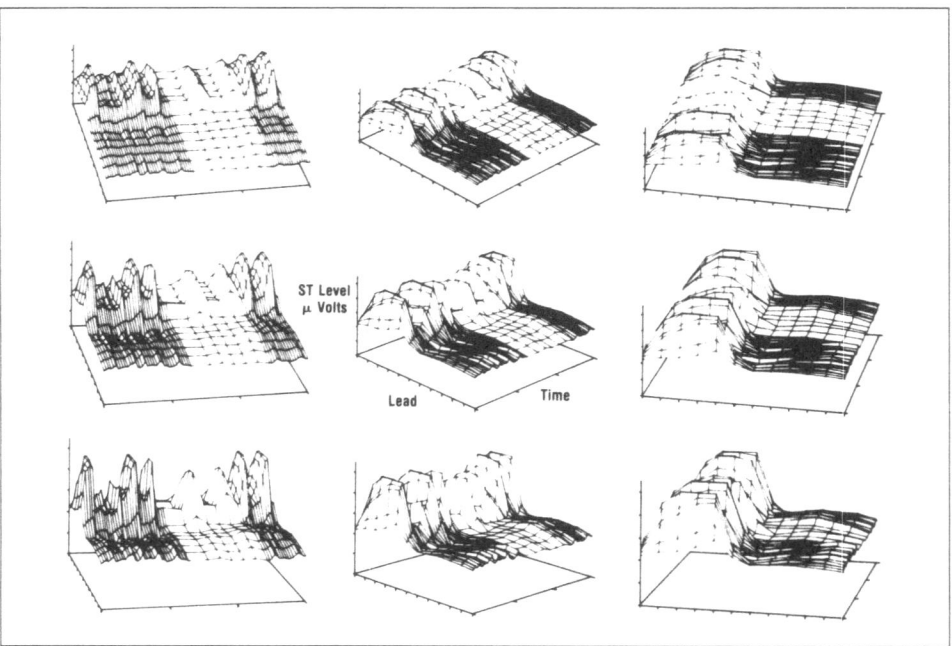

Fig. 3. Graphic output from 12-lead ST monitor during nine balloon inflations in LAD-diagonal bifurcation lesion, showing anterior elevation and reciprocal inferior depression reproduced with repeated occlusions despite variation in amplitude of ST deviation; b) output of same study rotated in three-dimensional space to favor appreciation of temporal (episode duration, lower left) or precordial (lower right) characteristics. (Reprinted with permission from [23]).

100

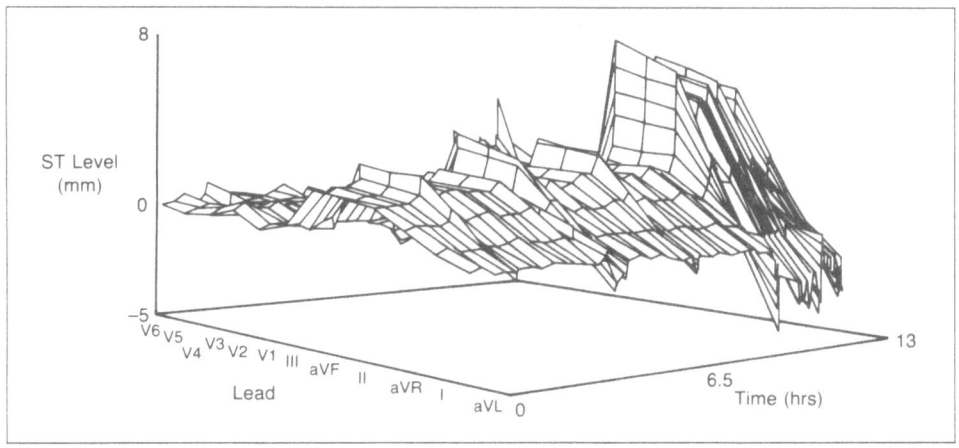

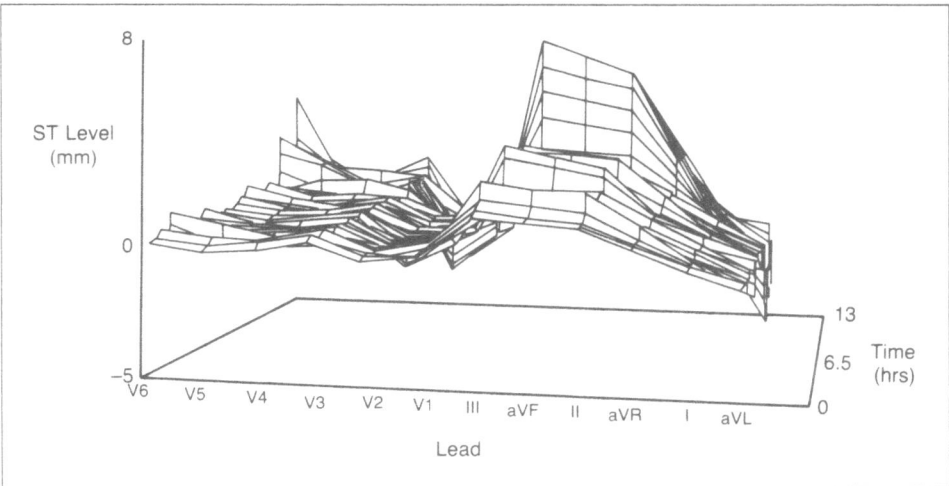

Fig. 4. Graphic output from 12-lead ST monitor in patient awaiting PTCA of residual stenosis in the RCA following successful thrombolytic therapy. During the night, the heavily sedated patient slept; monitor detected three transient episodes of ischemia, then a fourth more severe and persistent episode, all characterized by inferior ST elevation with lateral extension and reciprocal anterior ST depression. Catheterization disclosed total occlusion of the RCA. The patient had to be awakened for the procedure, and was asymptomatic throughout.

in the reference fingerprint pattern showed a clear hierarchy of multilead ST activity that could effectively focus attention to high risk patients even in the absence of symptoms. Of the 524 patients monitored after angiographically successful elective or emergency intracoronary interventions, 18 % (92) had transient ST episodes during their CCU stay. Patients with no ST episodes had a 1 % incidence of untoward clinical events (MI, urgent bypass, sudden death, or death) compared to a 28 %

incidence in patients with ST episodes. Of the patients with ST episodes, 57 % had only ST depression over all leads recorded, while 43 % had ST elevation in at least one lead. Patients with ST depression only had a 2 % incidence of clinical endpoints, compared to a 65 % incidence among patients with ST elevation. Patients with ST elevation in the CCU in a pattern different from the precordial "fingerprint" obtained during each patient's PTCA or acute MI experienced untoward clinical outcomes in 14 %, while 88 % of patients with a fingerprint match had untoward endpoints. All ST hierarchy subgroup comparisons (no ST episodes vs any ST episodes, ST depression vs ST elevation, and ST elevation different from fingerprints vs ST elevation pattern same as the fingerprint) were significant.

While most of our patients were recorded during and after elective PTCA, two of the 92 patients with ST episodes in the CCU presented in the early stages (< 3 h) of acute Q-wave infarction. In each of these patients, despite the evolution of QRS changes on the resting ECG, angiographically documented reocclusion of the infarct vessel still reproduced the initially documented precordial ST fingerprint pattern.

Of the 92 patients with transient ischemia in the CCU after intracoronary intervention, standard clinical CCU surveillance would have underestimated or missed ischemic episodes in 78 %: 28 % who had only silent episodes; 23 % with mixed silent and symptomatic episodes; and 27 % who had more than 15 min of markedly abnormal ST deviation prior to the onset of symptoms. Untoward clinical events were seen in a significant number of these patients, including total coronary occlusion and "silent" MI in four patients, and more than 15 min of marked ST deviation preceding MI with sudden death in two patients and MI with subsequent patient death in two patients.

Dicussion

ST analysis focused on quantification of "total ischemic burden" over the recording period is generally examined with regard to number of episodes, duration of episodes, and severity of ST displacement in the lead examined. Application of these largely arbitrary parameters has ignored important variables such as the presence of ST elevation vs ST depression and the number and location of leads active over the precordium. ST elevation and precordial lead activity, documented in the unstable angina and infarction literature as prognosticators [26, 27] and frequently used as trial entry criteria in studies of thrombolysis [4—11], historically were omitted from ST segment monitoring investigations because of the technical limitations of available devices. These technical limitations have now been overcome, allowing more comprehensive approaches to characterization of transient ischemia.

Continuous ST segment monitoring in patients with coronary artery disease has been repeatedly shown to identify periods of transient myocardial ischemia in the absence of symptoms [12—17]. While prognosis in some patient subgroups has been related to total ischemic burden as determined with ST monitoring [28] and while medical therapy has been shown to alter frequency and severity of ST episodes on Holter [17], more aggressive, invasive therapy in the absence of clinical symptoms has remained controversial. With the ever more widespread use of thrombolytic therapy and PTCA for non-surgical revascularization in both emergency and elective situations, the importance of this controversy will continue to grow. On the one hand, it is quite clear that occlusion of an unstable coronary site can occur prior to or in the complete absence of patient symptoms, and still result later in severe pump dysfunction, life-threatening arrhythmias, and death. On the other hand, aggressive therapies with attendant costs and risks must be considered cautiosly in asymptomatic patients who have had an angiographically apparently successful intracoronary intervention.

Transient episodes of ST segment deviation per se, while associated with a significantly higher complication rate than in patients with no such deviation after non-surgical revascularization (28 % vs 1 %, respectively) are, in our opinion, too non specific to independently merit aggressive therapy in asymptomatic patients. Of patients with ST deviation, the presence of ST elevation was significantly more specific than the presence of ST depression alone (65 % vs 2 %, respectively). In our experience, adequate assurance that ST depression in one or more leads is primary and not reciprocal to ST elevation occurring simultaneously elsewhere on the precordium requires monitoring of a minimum of three leads addressing anterior, inferior, and lateral electrical vectors [20—22]. Thus, ST depression alone also does not, based on our data, support more aggressive therapy in an asymptomatic patient after intracoronary intervention. ST depression in patients who manifest only ST depression during their reference event, ie., patients who have reference ST fingerprints that show only ST depression (as is not uncommon in patients with circumflex coronary occlusion), and/or patients who have severe symptoms associated with ST depression, may need more individualized consideration regarding risks/benefits of more aggressive or invasive therapy.

Patients with ST elevation in precordial areas different from their reference ST fingerprints have a significantly higher complication rate than patients with no ST changes (14 % vs 1 %, respectively), but probably include patients who manifest non-ischemic transient ST elevation from early repolarization or from the small positional changes that occur even in patients at bedrest. Again, our data would suggest that this is not a population who, if asymptomatic, would be likely to benefit from aggressive therapy. On the other hand, patients whose coronary sites transition from the relative stability of a successful intervention as angiographically assessed in the catheterization laboratory to instability that leads to clinical morbidity and mortality in the CCU are sensitively and specifically identified with multi-lead continuous ST segment monitoring when ST elevation is compared to their own reference event ST fingerprint. Of our patients, 88 % with ST elevation in the CCU who had recurrence of their ST fingerprint pattern had a morbid event, regardless of the presence or absence of clinical symptoms. This pattern was seen to recur even when events were markedly different in amplitude of ST deviation (Figs. 1—4), and even with the evolution of Q-waves in patients with successful early reperfusion during acute MI. It has thus become our standard clinical practice to proceed with aggressive anti-ischemic, anti-platelet, and anti-coagulant therapy, and even return to the cardiac catheterization laboratory with a completely asymptomatic patient in the face of recurrence and persistence of the reference ST fingerprint pattern on the bedside continuous ST segment monitor.

The surface electrocardiographic signal is a relatively crude summation of electrical vectors that does not elucidate pathophysiologic mechanisms but, rather, reflects alterations in the common end pathway of myocardial ischemia. For all its crudity, however, microprocessor-based signal acquisition and processing allow such comprehensive and virtually instantaneous waveform analysis on a continuous basis that use of the patient as his/her own reference, both as baseline and as coronary occlusion "fingerprint" template, is possible. As our data show, the clinical relevance of this distinction almost triples the specificity of ST segment changes for detection of an unstable coronary site, with no detectable loss of sensitivity. Moreover, this practical, noninvasive technology is an adjunct to, but independent of, angiographic/anatomic appearance of the intervention site in the cath lab or the report of subjective patient symptoms in the CCU environment.

References

1. Dorros G, Cowley MJ, Sinpson J, Bentivoglio LG, Block PC, Bourassa M, Detre K, Gosselin AJ, Gruntzig AR, Kelsey SF, Kent KM, Mock MB, Mullin SM, Myler RK, Passamani ER, Stertzer SH, Williams DO (1983) Percutaneous transluminal coronary angioplasty: report of complications from the National Heart, Lung, and Blood Institute PTCA Registry. Circulation 67: 723–730
2. Cowley M, Dorros G, Kelsey S, Raden M, Detre M (1984) Acute coronary events associated with percutaneous transluminal coronary angioplasty. Am J Cardiol 53: 12C–16C
3. Bredlau CE, Roubin GS, Leimgruber PP, Douglas JS Jr., King SB III, Gruentzig AR (1985) In-hospital morbidity and mortality in patients undergoing elective coronary angioplasty. Circulation 72: 1044–1052
4. Chesebro JH, Knatterud G, Roberts R, Borer J, Cohen LS, Dalen J, Dodge HT, Francis CK, Hillis D, Ludbrook P, Markis JE, Mueller H, Passamani ER, Powers ER, Rao AK, Robertson T, Ross A, Ryan TJ, Sobel BE, Willerson J, Williams DO, Zaret BL, Braunwald E (1987) Thrombolysis in myocardial infarction (TIMI) trial, phase I: a comparison between intravenous tissue plasminogen activator and intravenous streptokinase. Circulation 76: 142–154
5. Topol EJ, George BS, Kereiakes DJ, Candela RJ, Abbottsmith CW, Stump DC, Boswick JM, Stack RS, Califf RM, and the TAMI Study Group (1988) Comparison of two dose regimens of intravenous tissue plasminogen activator for acute myocardial infarction. Am J Cardiol 61: 723–728
6. Brower RW, Arnold AER, Lubsen J, Verstraete M, on behalf of the European Cooperative Study Group (1988) Coronary patency after intravenous infusion of recombinant tissue-type plasminogen activator in acute myocardial infarction. JACC 11: 681–688
7. Harrison DG, Ferguson DW, Collins SM, Skorton DJ, Ericksen EE, Kioschos JM, Marcus ML, White CW (1984) Rethrombosis after reperfusion with streptokinase: importance of geometry of residual lesions. Circulation 69: 991–999
8. Gold HK, Leinback RC, Garabedian HD, Yasuda T, Johns JA, Grossbard EB, Palacios I, Collen D (1986) Acute coronary reocclusion after thrombolysis with recombinant human tissue-type plasminogen activator: prevention by a maintenance infusion. Circulation 73: 347–352
9. Hays LJ, Beller GA, Moore CA, Burwell LR, Craddock GB, Gascho JA, Smucker ML, Tedesco C, Nygaard TW (1988) Short-term infarct vessel patency with aspirin and dipyridamole started 24 to 36 hours after intravenous streptokinase. Am Heart Jnl 115: 717–721
10. Schroder R, Neuhans KL, Linderer T, Leizorovicz A, Wegscheider K, Tebbe U for the ISAM study group (1987) Risk of death from recurrent ischemic events after intravenous streptokinase in acute myocardial infarction: results from the Intravenous Streptokinase in Myocardial Infarction (ISAM) study. Circulation 76 (suppl II): 44–51
11. Gash AK, Spann JF, Sherry S, Belber AD, Carabello BA, McDonough MT, Mann RH, McCann WE, Gault JH, Gentzler RD, Kent RL (1986) Factors influencing reocclusion after coronary thrombolysis for acute myocardial infarction. Am J Cardiol 57: 175–177

12. Stern S, Tzivoni D (1974) Early detection of silent ischemic heart disease by 24-hour electrocardiographic monitoring of active subjects. Br Heart J 36: 481—486
13. Deanfield JE, Selwyn AP, Chierchia S, Maseri A, Riberio P, Krikler S, Morgan M (1983) Myocardial ischaemia during daily life in patients with stable angina: its relation to symptoms and heart rate changes. Lancet 1: 753—758
14. Deanfield JE, Shea M, Ribiero P, de Landsheere CM, Wilson RA, Horlock P, Selwyn AP (1984) Transient ST-segment depression as a marker of myocardial ischemia during daily life. Am J Cardiol 54: 1195—1200
15. Schang SJ, Pepine CJ (1977) Transient asymptomatic ST segment depression during daily activity. Am J Cardiol 39: 396—402
16. Biagini A, Mazzei MG, Carpeggiani C, Testa R, Antonelli R, Michelassi C, L'Abbate A, Maseri A (1982) Vasospastic ischemic mechanism of frequent asymptomatic transient ST-T changes during continuous electrocardiographic monitoring in selected unstable angina patients. Am Heart J 103: 13—19
17. Imperi GA, Lambert CR, Coy K, Lopez L, Pepine CJ (1987) Effects of titrated beta blockade (metoprolol) on silent myocardial ischemia in ambulatory patients with coronary artery disease. Am J Cardiol 60: 519—524
18. Krucoff MW, Green CE, Satler LF, Miller FC, Pallas RS, Kent KM, Del Negro AA, Pearle DL, Fletcher RD, Rackley CE (1986) Noninvasive detection of coronary artery patency using continuous ST-segment monitoring. Am J Cardiol 57: 916—922
19. Davies GJ, Chierchia S, Maseri A (1984) Prevention of myocardial infarction by very early treatment with intracoronary streptokinase: some clinical observations. N Engl J Med 311: 1488—1492
20. Krucoff MW, Pope JE, Bottner RK, Renzi RH, Wagner GS, Kent KM (1987) Computer-Assisted ST-segment Monitoring: Experience During and after brief coronary occlusion. J Electrocardiology Suppl 15—21
21. Krucoff MW, Akbari MM, Stark KS, Ahmed SW, Parente AR, Renzi RH, Kent KM. Pitfalls of 1 and 2 lead ST segment recording of silent or sysmptomatic ischemia. Circulation (abstr), in press
22. Krucoff, MW (1988) Identification of high-risk patients with silent myocardial ischemia after percutaneous transluminal coronary angioplasty by multilead monitoring. Am J Cardiol 61: 29F-34F
23. Krucoff MW, Pope JE, Bottner RK, Adams IM, Wagner GS, Kent KM (1987) "Dedicated ST-segment monitoring in the CCU after successful coronary angioplasty: incidence and prognosis of silent and symptomatic ischemia" in Silent Ischemia, von Arnim Th, Maseri A eds., Steinkopff Verlag, Darmstadt, p. 140—146
24. Krucoff MW, Parente AR, Bottner RK, Renzi RH, Stark KS, Shugoll RA, Ahmed SW, De-Michele J, Stroming SL, Green CE, Rackley CE, Kent KM (1988) Stability of multilead ST-segment "fingerprints" over time after percutaneous transluminal coronary angioplasty and its usefulness in detecting reocclusion. Am J Cardiol 61: 1232—1237
25. Adams IM, Mortara DW (1987) "A new method for electrocardiographic monitoring" in Acute Coronary Care 1987, Califf RM and Wagner GS eds., Martinus Nijhoff, Boston 1987, p. 165—176
26. Severi S, Marraccini P, Michelassi C, Orsini E, Nassisi V, L'Abbate A (1988) Electrocardiographic manifestations and in-hospital prognosis of transient acute myocardial ischemia at rest. Am J Cardiol 61: 31—37
27. Johnson SM, Mauritson DR, Winiford MD, Willerson JT, Firth BG, Cary JR, Hillis LD (1982) Continuous electrocardiographic monitoring in patients with unstable angina pectoris: identification of high-risk subgroup with severe coronary disease, variant angina, and/or impaired early prognosis. Am Heart J 103: 4—12
28. Gottlieb SO, Weisfeldt ML, Ouyang P (1986) Silent ischemia as a marker for early unfavorable outcomes in patients with unstable angina. N Engl J Med 314: 1214—1219

Authors' address:
Mitchell W. Krucoff, M.D.
Duke University Medical Center
Erwin Road
Durham, NC 27710
USA

Discussion

VON ARNIM:

Do you have the possibility to see all those nice "fingerprint" pictures over all leads and over a length of time already in real time?

KRUCOFF:

In real time the ST deviation over 12 leads is summated as a single line trend. That is visualized on the LCD screen on the device at bed side. The multi-color pictures are only from the connection to an IBM PC.

VON ARNIM:

I think the main advantage of this device is that you have its information at the bedside in real time. What you are showing goes beyond that and the work with the PC is an interesting scientific aside to it, however less useful yet for patient care.

CHIERCHA:

Do you have any validation of the alarm system, in other words do you have a simultaneous recording of digital data on the box, as well as analogoue data on the 12-lead ECG continuously to see whether the box triggers properly?

KRUCOFF:

There are two sides to that answer. We did 150 consecutive patients with simultaneous 3-channel Holter recording. Now, that is not as straightforward a validation as it sounds; as you know, for Holter ECG we use bipolar ECG vectors and the amplitudes, are different at baseline, with a bipolar relative to 12 standard lead vector. However, the correlation between those two in terms of unequivocal events was almost 100 %. The box with 12 leads still does get some high lateral areas that, at least our 3 Holter vectors do not capture. For all the digital trends you can bring up just the ECG information itself and inspect it visually. That is the other side of the validation. Every time the box triggers, we just print out the ECGs and read them. The box is by design made to be overly sensitive rather than overly specific. It has incorporated signal processing which comes from the case exercise ECG system, so it deals with noise in a very robust way electrically. Nontheless, there are triggers for noise or for artefact that do require real time interaction, so the device is made to be overly sensitive rather than specific.

Holter-monitoring for detecting silent ischemia

D. Andresen, Th. Brüggemann, and R. Schröder

Department of Cardiology, Klinikum Steglitz, Freie Universität Berlin, FRG

Introduction

Holter-monitoring has been suggested for detecting transient coronary ischemia [1, 2, 7, 9, 12, 13, 16]. Early investigation used frequency-modulated recording systems for ST-segment analysis. The application of direct-recording systems was limited because of the inadequate low-frequency response, which may leas to inaccurae ST-segment recordings [3, 4, 17]. Today, some direct-recording systems have characteristics that seem to make these devices suitable for detecting ST-segment changes [6, 10, 15]. But it is still unclear how accurately ST-segment alterations can be detected with the different systems. We investigated the direct-recording Holter-monitoring systems CardioData Mk4 with recorder PR3, CardioData Mk4 with Spacelabs recorder, DMI Eclipse with DMI recorder, Reynolds Pathfinder II with Oxford replay PB2 and recorder MR-10, Reynolds Pathfinder III with Tracker and Marquett, in comparison to a standard ECG recorder Picker Schwarzer C6800.

The investigation consisted of the following three steps:
1) Measurements of amplitude and phase response;
2) Measurement of the accuracy of computer-produced ST-segment depressions;
3) Analyzing the accuracy of exercised-induced ST-segment depression.

Methods and results

Amplitude and phase response

The transmission quality of a system can be assessed by determining the frequency curve of the amplitude. We used sinus waves of different frequencies, which were produced by a function generator (Wavetek 117) and had an amplitude of 2 mV. In order to determine how the device influenced the amplitude of the sinus wave at a given frequency we calculated the difference between the amplitude of the input and output signal. If the ratio between the output and input amplitude is 0 dB, no distortion of the signal by the device has occurred. A ratio of > 0 dB indicates that the signal has been artificially amplified, while a ratio of < 0 dB shows that the signal has been attenuated by the device. A deviation of $\pm$ dB from the zero line was tolerated, regarding a frequency curve as linear.

The recorded sinus waves were fed into the Holter-monitoring system, and an example of each frequency was printed out. The ratio of the output to the input amplitude was then plotted on logarithmic paper.

A phase-sensitive signal was used to determine the phase response. The relative phase response was calculated as $f(t = \sin Lt + \sin 3\,Lt$.

With the aid of the function generator, the test signal with a peak-to-peak amplitude of 2 mV ranging in frequency from 0.05—10 Hz was applied to the input of the different recording systems. The quality of the input signal was monitored by an oscilloscope (Tektronix 5103N). The interval between two peaks of the same polarity was standardized to the total amplitude of the signal and plotted on semilogarithmic paper.

The amplitude and phase responses of the different systems are shown in Figs. 1 and 2. All longterm ECG-recording systems markedly differed from the standard ECG recorder with respect to the amplitude response. But there were also differences between the various Holter-monitoring systems both with respect to the lower frequency limit of −3 dB and the linearity of the curve. The relative phase shift likewise differed from one system to the next (Fig. 2).

Measurement of the accuracy of computer-induced ST-segment depressions

In order to determine the distortion of ST-segments by different Holter-systems, a standard ECG signal was produced by the function generator. Different degrees of horizontal ST-segment depressions ranging from 0.05—0.5 mV were generated. The corresponding ECG was recorded over a period of 20 min, and examples of the different ST-segment depressions were printed out by the analyzer during assessment. Nominal and actual values were plotted against each other.

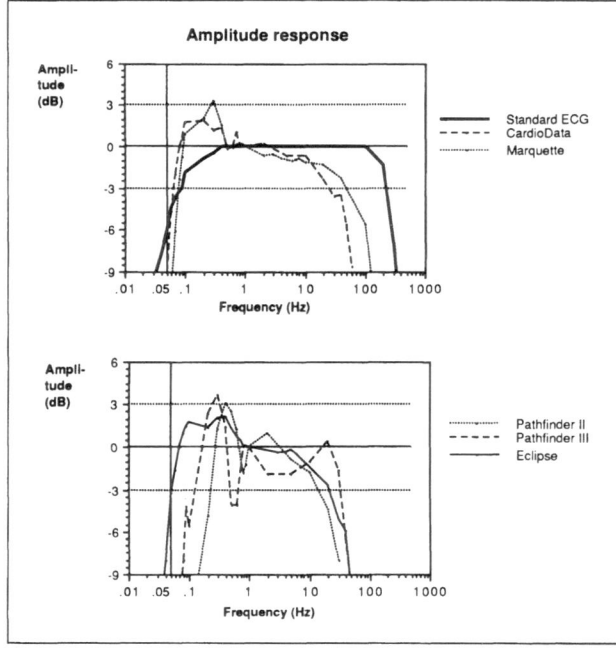

Fig. 1. Amplitude vs frequency response curves derived from input sinus waves ranging from 0.01 to 500 Hz. x-axis: frequency (Hz) in logarithmic sacale; axis. ratio of Vout/Vin (dB). Hz = Hertz, V = Amplitude, dB = Decibel. For standard ECG the low and high frequency cut-off point (−3dB) was found at 0.09 and 220 Hz, respectively.

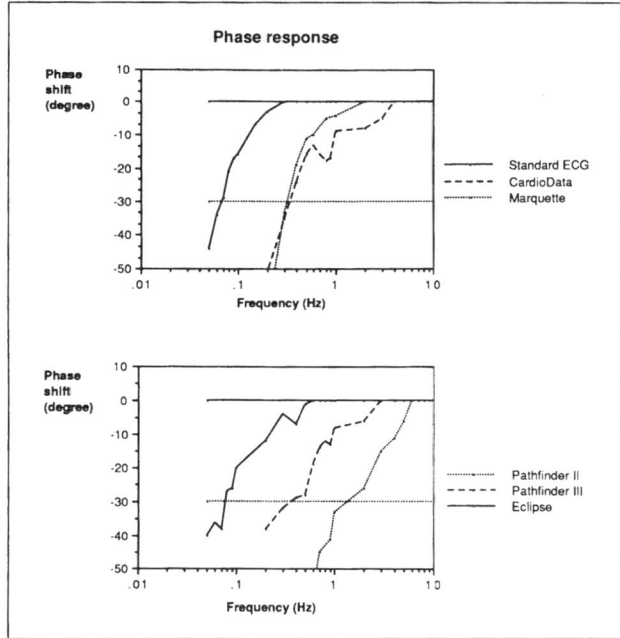

Fig. 2. Phase response curves produced with a phase-sensitive waveform at a frequency range from 0.05 to 10 Hz.

For standard ECG a phase shift at −30 degree was detected at 0.07 Hz, while for the Holter-systems these points were found quite earlier.

Figure 3 shows examples of the original recordings of some longterm monitoring systems to which an input signal with an ST-segment depression of 0.3 mV was applied. Figure 4 demonstrates the extent of horizontal ST-segment depression for the different test signals with the corresponding ST-segment depression as recorded by the systems investigated. While the standard ECG recorder produces a curve that runs exactly along the identity line (the ST-segment depression registered by the ECG recorder is identical to the ST-segment depression applied), some Holter-monitoring systems showed deviations.

Analyzing the accuracy of exercise-induced ST-segment depression

Our purpose was to estimate the reliability of direct-recording Holter-systems for the detection of exercise-induced ST-segment depressions found with standard ECG-recorder during submaximal stress-testing. We investigated 22 patients (seven female, 15 male) ranging in age from 46 to 78 years with a mean of 57 years. All patients had stable angina pectoris and a positive exercise stress test with an ST-segment depression of > 0.1 mV in at least two precordial leads. No patient had a bundle-branch block or cardiac pacemaker. All patients underwent a second, symptom-limited bicycle exercise test in a supine position according to the Bruce protocol (with simultaneous Holter-monitoring and standard ECG registration).

We used a six-channel standard ECG recorder (Picker Schwarzer C6800) allowing the registration of 12 leads. Electrodes were positioned to record the limb leads (I,

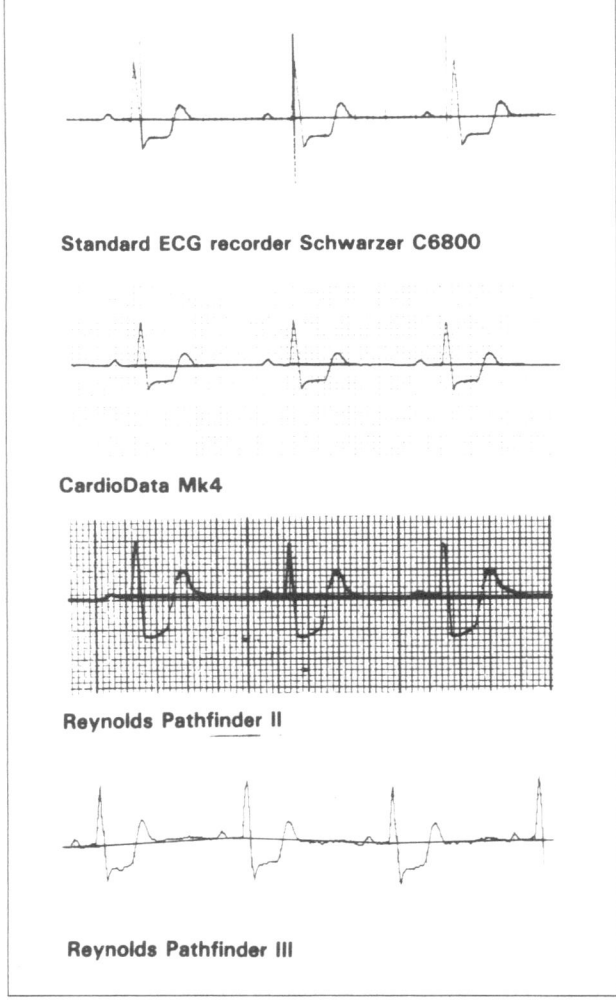

Fig. 3. Alteration of an ECG-signal with a strict horizonal ST-segment depression of 0.3 mV (= 3mm).

Standard ECG recorder Schwarzer C6800

CardioData Mk4

Reynolds Pathfinder II

Reynolds Pathfinder III

II, III, aVR, aVL and aVF) as well as the precordial leads (V1—V6) in the usual way.

A CardioData PR3 recorder with two bipolar leads (LEG 1 and 2) was used as a test of a longterm ECG system. The two exploratory electrodes were attached to V5/V6 and xiphoid locations. The two negative electrodes were positioned ad the upper sternum (Fig. 5).

Symptom-limited bicycle exercise testing in a supine position was performed according to the Bruce protocol [5]. During the stress test and subsequent recovery period, the 12-lead ECG and the two longterm ECG leads were recorded every minute with the standard ECG recorder using a special swith device (Fig. 5). Simultaneously, the two longterm ECG leads were recorded with a longterm ECG cassette recorder.

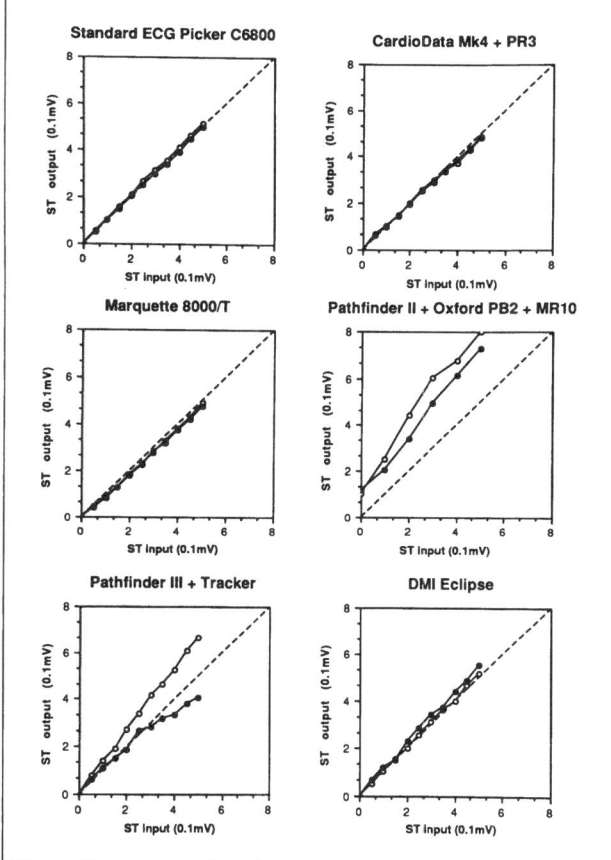

Fig. 4. Accuracy of detection computer-produced ST-segment depressions (○———○ = lead 1, ●———● = lead 2).

During tape analysis with the computer system, a 10-s sample from both leads was printed out at one-min intervals. The ST-segment changes were measured by hand, taking the average of five segments.

The two longterm ECG leads presented on the standard ECG were compared to the two leads presented on the longterm ECG. This comparison was made with regard to the beginning, time of maximal depression, and the maximal extent of ST-segment changes.

Figure 6 shows the time intervals between the different leads. Good agreement was found between the corresponding leads LEG 1 — ECG 1 and LEG 2 — ECG 2. Only lead LEG 2 showed a slight deviation. The time of the maximal ST-segment depression was detected one min earlier than in lead ECG 2.

The maximal extent of ST-segment depression is shown in Fig. 7 for lead 1 and in Fig. 8 for lead 2. The good agreement in the entire patient group could also be confirmed for the individual patient. Differences were, however, observed in some cases.

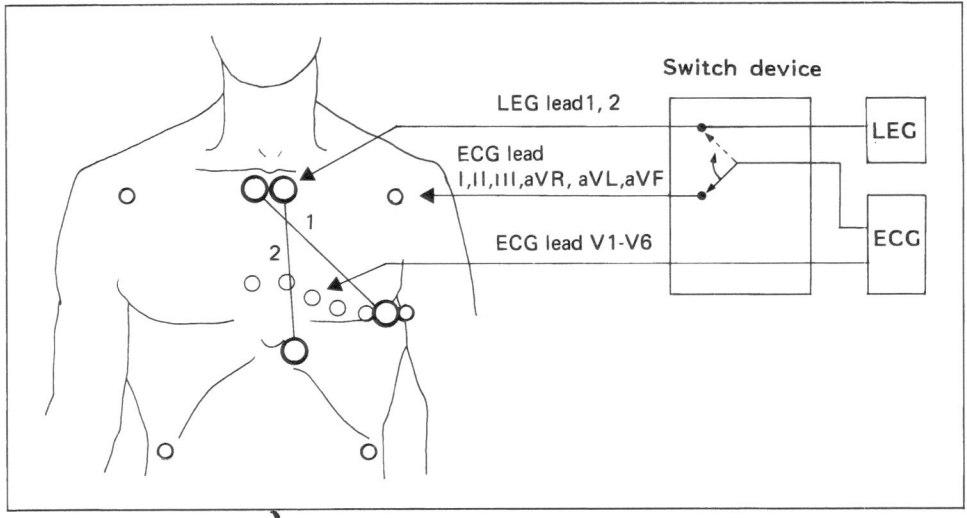

Fig. 5. Simultaneous registration of the 12-lead standard ECG and the bipolar leads of the longterm ECG.

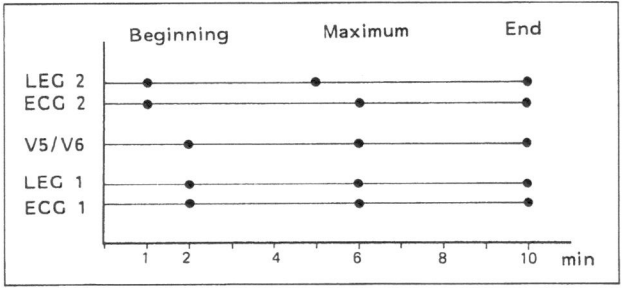

Fig. 6. Beginning, time of maximum, and end of ST-segment depression (median values) found with the standard ECG and longterm ECG.

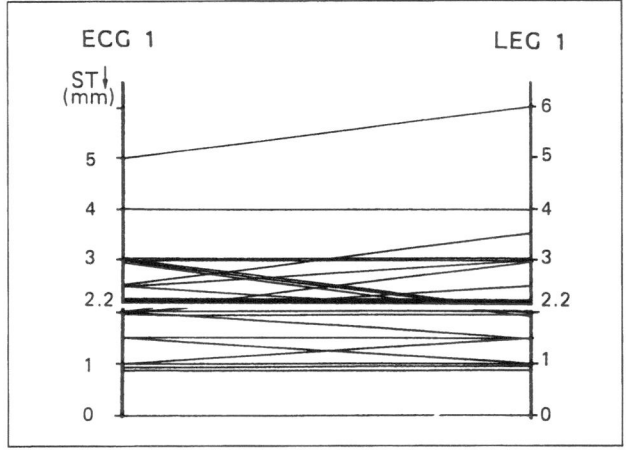

Fig. 7. Maximal extent of ST-segment depression found with a standard ECG (lead ECG 1) in comparison to the longterm ECG (lead LEG 1).

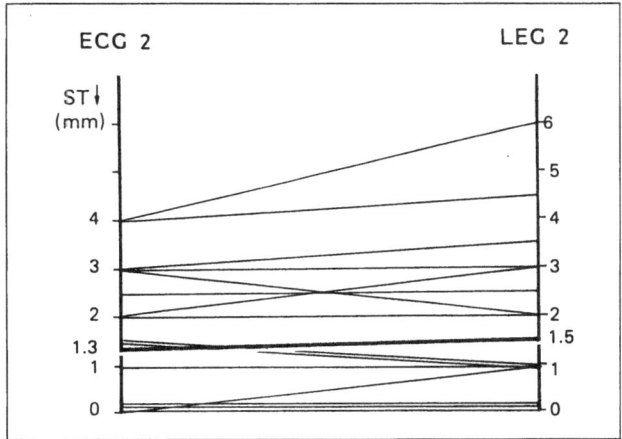

Fig. 8. Maximal extent of ST-segment depression found with a standard ECG (lead ECG 2) in comparison to the longterm ECG (lead LEG 2).

Discussion

In 1966, Berson and Pipberger [3] investigated the influence of the filter slope and frequency limit of an ECG amplifier on ST-segment recording. The concluded from their results that in order to assure a high accuracy of ST-segment recording a lower frequency limit of 0.05 Hz at a filter slope of 6 dB per octave was necessary.

On the basis of these results, the American Heart Association requested a lower heart rate limit of 0.05 Hz both for standard ECG recorders [11] and longterm devices [14]. However, the reproduction quality of a longterm ECG recorder is decisively influenced by the behavior of the ECG amplifier over the entire frequency range. In addition, frequency curve measurements should not be limited to the recording device, as it is frequently done by the manufacturers, but they should include the entire system (recorder, replay unit, analyzer and printer).

Various procedures are available for determining the phase response [8, 18, 19]. We used the method of Wagner [19]. Trompler et al. [18], who used a comparable method to measure phase shifts in two longterm recording systems obtained similar results. The results reported by Taylor and Vincent [17] suggest that distortion of the ST-segment in longterm ECG recording is mainly caused by a poor phase curve. Figure 9 shows how a phase shift alone can influence the accuracy of ST-segment recording. A horizontally depressed ST-segment is more and more obliterated as the phase shift increases and finally takes an ascending course.

The reliability of a longterm ECG system in the detection of myocardial ischemia can only be investigated by comparison with a system that has a proven capacity for detecting myocardial ischemia. We therefore chose a standard six-channel ECG recorder routinely used for the ECG registration during exercise stress tests. Comparison of the maximal extent of ST-segment depression revealed a good correlation between the corresponding leads. Nevertheless, differences were observed in indi-

113

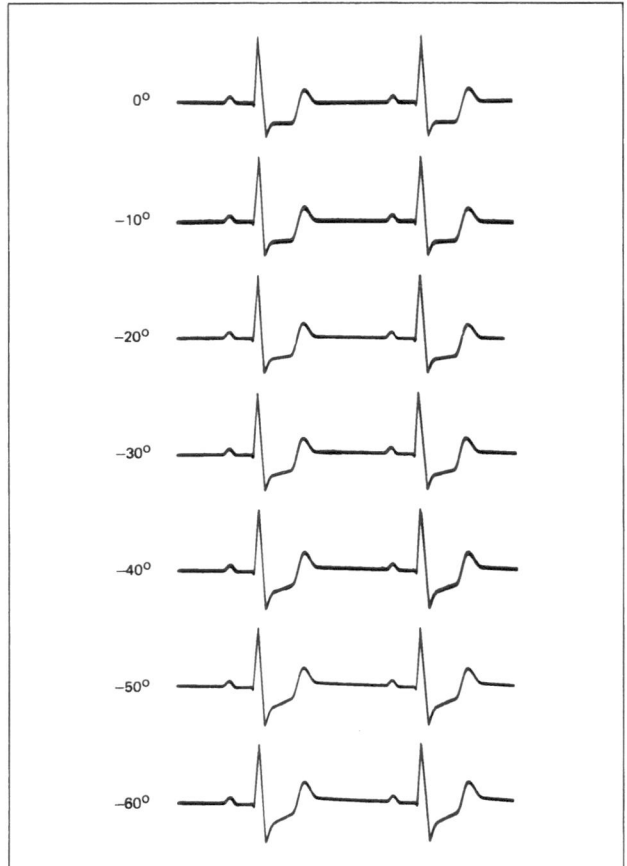

Fig. 9. Influence of the phase shift of different degrees on the ST-segment. A horizontally depressed ST-segment is more and more obliterated as the phase shift increases and finally takes an ascending course.

vidual patients. This might be due to inaccuracies during measurement: the J-point was more difficult to define on the longterm ECG strip than on the chart of the standard ECG recorder. The J-point represents a change of the frequency contents from higher to lower frequency components in the ECG [4]. The limited high-frequency response of Holter-monitoring systems may lead to an inaccurate beginning of the ST-segment. Thus, the ST-segment depression could not always be measured at identical positions in the longterm- and standard-ECG on the basis of our study; it is not possible to decide which of the longterm ECG recording systems investigated should be preferred for the diagnosing of ST-segment alterations. Many factors, such as the quality of the recorded ECG, temporal resolution of the depicted trend, velocity of analysis, easy operation of the system, and accuracy in analyzing arrhythmias, have to be taken into consideration. But we think that the measurements we performed should be made a prerequisite for any system that is offered for ST-segment analysis.

Conclusions

Direct-recording Holter-monitoring systems, like frequency-modulated devices, are basically able to faithfully represent ST-segment depressions. Data on the lower frequency limit are not sufficient. Besides the measurement of amplitude and phase curves, the reliability of detecting ST-segment alterations should be checked using standardized test signals. The reliability in detecting myocardial ischemias induced by exercise stress-testing could be the last step of testing Holter-systems, before they are used in clinical practice.

References

1. von Arnim Th, Höfling B, Schreiber M (1985) ST-Segment-Analyse im Langzeit-EKG. Deutsch Med Wschr 26: 1047—1051
2. Balasubramanian V, Lahiri A, Green HL, Stott FD, Raftery EB (1986) Ambulatory ST-segment monitoring, problems, pitfalls, solutions and clinical implications. Br Heart J 44: 419
3. Berson AS, Pipberger HV (1966) The low frequency response of electrocardiographs: a frequent source of recording errors. Am Heart J 71: 779
4. Bragg-Ramschel DA, Anderson CA, Winkle RA (1982) Frequency response characteristics of ambulatory ECG monitoring systems and their implication for ST-segment analysis. Amer Heart J 103: 419
5. Bruce RA (1971) Exercise testing of patients with coronary heart disease: principles and normal standards for evaluation. Ann Clin Res 3: 323—332
6. Brüggemann Th, Andresen D, Erbherr G, Schröder R (1987) Frequency response characteristics of long-term ECG systems in comparison to a standard ECG recorder. Europ Heart J 8 Suppl 2: 183
7. Deanfield J, Maseri A, Selwyn A (1983) Myocardial ischemia during daily life in patients with stable angina: Its relation to symptoms and heart rate changes. Lancet: 753—758
8. Frey AW, Brose JW, Flachenecker G, Theisen K (1988) Stumme Myokardischämie im Langzeit-EKG: Ist der Standard der American Heart Association für die ST-Segment-Analyse ausreichend? Z Kardiol 77: 110—114
9. Gallino A, Chierchia, S, Smith G, Croom M, Morgan M, Marchesi C, Maseri A (1984) Computer system for analysis of ST-segment changes on 24 hour Holter monitoring tapes: comparison with other available systems. J Amer Coll Cardiol 4: 245
10. Imperi GA, Lambert CR, Pepine CJ (1986) Low frequency requirements for reproduction of ischemic ST-segment abnormalities during activity in man. J Amer Coll Cardiol 7,2: 104A
11. Pipberger HV, Arzbaecher RC, Berson AS, Briller SA, Brody DA, Flowers NC, Geselowitz DB, Lepeschkin E, Oliver GC, Schmitt OH, Spach M (1975) Recommendations for standardization of leads and specifications for instruments in electrocardiology and vectorcardiography. Report of the Committee on Electrocardiography. American Heart Association. Circulation 52: 11—31
12. Schang SJ, Pepine CJ (1977) Transient asymptomatic ST segment depression during daily activity. Am J Cardiol 39: 396—400
13. Selwyn AP, Fox K, Eves M, Oakley D, Dargie H, Schillingford J (1978) Myocardial ischemia in patients with frequent angina pectoris. Br Med J 2: 1594—1596
14. Sheffield LT, Berson A, Bragg-Remschel D, Gilette PC, Hermes RE, Hinkle L, Kennedy H, Mirvis DM, Oliver C (1985) Recommendations for standards of instrumentation and practice in the use of ambulatory electrocardiography. Report of the Committee on electrocardiography an cardiac electrophysiology, American Heart Association. Circulation 71: 3, 626a—636a
15. Shook TL, Balke CW, Kotilainen PW, Selwyn AP, Stone PH (1986) Accuracy of detection of myocardial ischemia by amplitude-modulated and frequency modulated Holter techniques. J Amer Coll Cardiol 7,2: 104 A

16. Stern S, Tzivioni D (19754) Early detection of silent ischemic heart disease by 24 hour elec-trocardiographic monitoring of active subjects. Br Heart J 36. 481—486
17. Taylor D, Vincent R (1983) Signal distortion in the electrocardiogram due to inadequate phase response. IEEE Trans Biom Engin 30: 352—356
18. Trompler AT, Horlamus R, Kreuzer H, Bethge KP (1987) ST-Segment Analyse mit dem Lang-zeit-EKG: Phasenlinearität verschiedener Systeme. Z Kardiol 76, Suppl 1: 90
19. Wagner JW (1979) A simple test for phase characteristics of chart recorders. IEEE Trans Biom Engin 26: 505—508

Author's address:
Priv.-Doz. Dr. med. D. Andresen
Klinikum Steglitz der FU
Med. Klinik und Poliklinik
Hindenburgdamm 30
1000 Berlin 45, FRG

Discussion

VON ARNIM:

What is the difference between the phase shifts at 0.08 Hz and 1.3 Hz? How does the frequency come into this phase shift problem?

ANDRESEN:

You can distinguish between measuring the phase shifts only in degrees. You can say the system has a phase shift up to 90 °, or you can say that the system has a phase shift of only 30 °. But you can also determine a normal range and say, up to a 30°-phase shift, is the normal range. Then you ask at which frequency this phase shift is really reached. The earlier this phase shift of 30 ° is reached, the more distortion of the ECG is expected.

Transient ischemic episodes — a marker for future cardiac events in patients with stable angina pectoris

Th. v. Arnim, U. Szeimies-Seebach, A. Erath, M. A. Schreiber and B. Höfling

Medizinische Klinik I und Institut für Med. Informationsverarbeitung, Statistik und Biomathematik, Ludwig-Maximilians-Universität, Klinikum Großhadern, Munich, FRG

Introduction

Coronary heart disease is the most frequent cause of death in industrialized countries. Besides its irreversible manifestations as myocardial infarction or sudden death, the disease presents itself in symptomatic form as angina pectoris or in asymptomatic form as silent ischemia. In recent years the similarities between silent and non-silent manifestations of transient ischemia have received much attention [1—4]. It has been shown that pain is not a very reliable warning system for patients with transient episodes of myocardial ischemia. Even in myocardial infarctions a high percentage of asymptomatic occurrences has been found [5].

For transient ischemic episodes, an importance can only be claimed as far, as there are prognostic implications. If silent ischemia is not a prognostic marker of more severe cardiac events to come, then it would not need to be treated. For patients who develop signs of electrocardiographic ischemia under exercise conditions, prognostic consequences of this finding have been shown in many studies [6—9]. With the more recent development of ambulatory electrocardiographic monitoring as a tool for the diagnosis of myocardial ischemia, several authors have demonstrated the prognostic significance of silent ischemic episodes in patients with unstable angina pectoris [10, 11, 12]. The prognostic implications of such episodes in patients with less severe and more stable forms of angina pectoris are less well established. We conducted a survey of patients with coronary angiography in our institution to demonstrate the prevalence of transient, predominantly silent ischemic episodes. These were patients with stable angina pectoris, and with a follow-up 4.5 years after the initial screening we investigated prognostic factors in these patients with special attention to the implications of initial ambulatory electrocardiographic monitoring.

Methods

Starting in January 1982, 306 patients who underwent coronary arteriography at our hospital were consecutively included in a study with 24-h-electrocardiographic monitoring, under the condition that the indication for the angiographic examination was coronary artery disease and not valvular heart disease or primary myocardial disease. Patients were excluded when they had bundle-branch-block or atrial fibrillation in the ECG or were on digitalis medication. This was done because of interference with the ST-segment analysis of the ECG [12a]. There were 249 males (81%, mean age 53 years, range 21–73 years) and 57 females (19%, mean age 54 years, range 38–69 years). At the initial examination data from the history of the patients about risk factors and concomitant diseases, resting and exercise ECG were all documented together with the results of the ambulatory electrocardiographic monitoring and coronary arteriography. Results of the initial examinations have been published previously [13, 14].

For the follow-up examination, data could be collected by repeat examinations, questionnaires, and telephone calls on 302 of 306 patients (98.7%). Present anginal status or the occurrence of cardiac events like coronary artery bypass graft operation, percutaneous transluminal coronary angioplasty, and acute myocardial infarction or death were recorded.

The results of the follow-up examinations were stored in the same data-bank as the initial data (Savod [15]) so that intercorrelations could be calculated. With the use of the BMDP statistical package [16], life-table analyses were performed and univariate comparisons were evaluated with the Mantel-Cox test. Multivariate step-wise regression analysis (Cox model) was done to identify independent prognostic influences of different variables.

Results

Of 302 patients on whom follow-up data were available, 25 (8.3%) had died during the follow-up period of 54.1 ± 3.6 months. Of those deaths, 20 (6.6%) were cardiac deaths. An acute myocardial infarction had occurred in 21 patients (7%) during the follow-up period. Thus the infarct-free survival of the total group was 86.4% over 4.5 years. Bypass operation was performed in 93 patients (30.8%) and PTCA in six patients (2.0%). If death, AMI, and revascularisation are taken together as cardiac events, 124 patients (40.7%) had a total of 140 cardiac events. These results of the follow-up examination were correlated with data from the initial examination on status of the coronary artery and results of ambulatory electrocardiographic monitoring. Of the 302 patients, 233 (77%) had significant coronary stenosis (≥ 70%) in at least one coronary artery. This was single-vessel disease in 56 patients, double-vessel disease in 61 patients, and triple-vessel disease in 116 patients. Of the 233 patients with significant coronary stenosis, 59 (25.3%) had transient ischemic episodes upon ambulatory electrocardiographic monitoring. These were defined as ST depression or elevation of at least 1 mm for more than one minute on dual channel, frequency modulated Holter monitoring, examined with visual analysis. Sixty-five percent of the transient ischemic episodes recorded with ambulatory monitoring were not accompanied by chest pain and/or anginal equivalents and were thus considered silent.

Figure 1 shows the life-table analysis of follow-up data on patients with single-, double-, or triple-vessel disease. The results are given for event-free-survival, where all events, i.e., revascularization, AMI, and death are counted. As would be expected, the survival curves separate according to the severity of vessel involvement.

Figure 2 shows survival curves for event-free-survial, as in Fig. 1, separated for severity of vessel involvement. For better clarity the curves for single- and double-

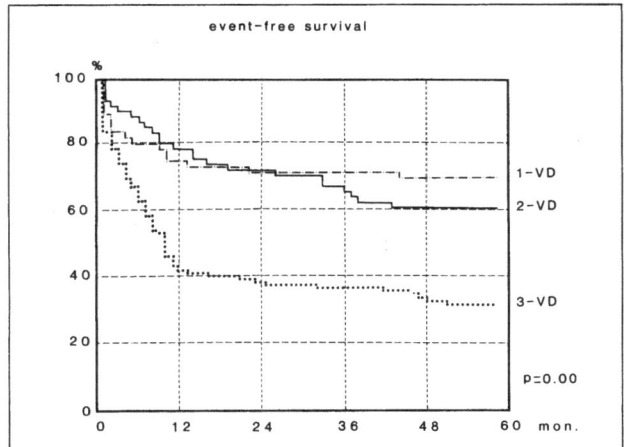

Fig. 1. Life-table analysis of survival on data of 302 patients 54 months (mean) after coronary angiography. In 233 patients with significant coronary stenosis an increased number of events (death, AMI, CABG or PTCA) is observed, which is highly significant for triple-vessel disease.

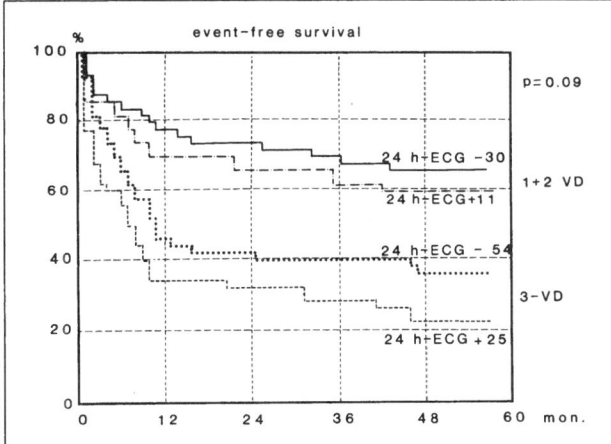

Fig. 2. Data on patients with significant coronary stenosis for event-free survival, similar to Fig. 1. In this figure the curves for single- and double-vessel disease, and for triple-vessel disease are separated according to the results of 24-h monitoring. In patients with transient ischemia on 24-h monitoring (24-h-ECG) the event-free survival is lower than in patients without transient ischemia. This separation shows a statistical trend (p = 0.09).

vessel disease are taken together. The curves for single-, double-vessel disease, and triple-vessel disease are separated according to the results of ambulatory electrocardiographic monitoring. It can be seen that over the course of the follow-up, patients who had shown transient ischemic episodes initially had a higher rate of subsequent cardiac events compared to patients without transient ischemic episodes. With the Mantel-Cox test, there is a trend towards statistically significant differences between patients with and without transient ischemic episodes.

The result of multivariate analysis with step-wise logistic regression are given in Table 1. With this result the different variables entered into the model can be tested for the independent prognostic information and each variable can contribute to the pronostication of the patient. The results given are for patients with documented significant coronary stenosis (n = 233). In step 0 on the lefthand side the variables

119

Table 1. Stepwise logistic regression (Cox model); All patients with significant CHD ($<75\%$ stenosis) n = 233; All cardiac events (death, n = 17/AMI, n = 21/CABG, n = 77/PTCA, n = 5).

Step 0			Step 1		
	x^2	p	(Gensini score removed)	x^2	p
1) Gensini score	45.037	0.000	1) ischemia on Holter	3.84	0.049
2) previous AMI	7.326	0.007	2) prompt NTG response	3.18	0.074
3) path. exercise	7.07	0.008	3) angina pectoris III/IV	2.47	0.116
4) prompt NTG response	5.19	0.023	4) hypertension	2.26	0.133
5) age	3.50	0.062	5) path. exercise	1.59	0.207
6) ischemia on Holter	3.16	0.076	6) age	1.23	0.268
7) male sex ·	2.15	0.143	7) male sex	0.43	0.513
8) ejection fraction	2.09	0.149	8) ejection fraction	0.31	0.575
9) hypertension	1.72	0.189	9) family history	0.08	0.772
10) angina pectoris III/IV	1.03	0.309	10) previous AMI	0.08	0.772
11) cholesterol	0.77	0.381	11) cholesterol	0.05	0.818
12) family history	0.76	0.383	12) smoking	0.02	0.885
13) smoking	0.17	0.683	13) diabetes	0.00	0.997
14) diabetes	0.03	0.857			

are given with their univariate values for Chi^2 statistic and univariate P-values. The severity of the coronary artery disease is quantified with the Gensini score. The Gensini score obviously has the highest impact on prognosis of the patients. In the first step of the multivariate stepwise regression analysis, the factor with the highest impact ist removed and the other factors are rearranged according to the independent prognostic information they can still provide. It is here that the results of the ambulatory electrocardiographic monitoring are the only variable that reaches statistical significance. All other factors show a very strong covariation with the degree of fixed coronary stenosis.

Discussion

The results of our study show that in patients with proven coronary artery disease, the presence of transient ischemic episodes on ambulatory monitoring is a marker for a subsequently increased rate of major cardiac events. As the prognostic implications remain significant, independent of the degree of fixed coronary stenosis, the occurrence of transient ischemia seems to convey some information on the activity of the ischemic heart disease over and above the degree of fixed narrowing of arteries.

However the results must be interpreted with caution regarding several special points in this study. The patient population was an obviously highly selective one: patients had been sent to the hospital because of complaints and previous disease and presented an accepted indication for coronary arteriography. Patients with unstable angina were excluded; however the patients were all more or less symptomatic around the time of the initial examination. Therefore the results of our study cannot be extrapolated to patients with completely silent ischemia. The patients in our study represent a sample of patients with symptomatic and asymptomatic ischemia, in whom the documented ischemic episodes were predominantly silent [14]. We are confident that patients such as those we studied appear frequently in clinical cardiology. Furthermore, we can be confident of the data because of a long follow-up period and an almost complete follow-up in a large group of patients. Information on prognostic implications of Holter monitoring in patients with stable angina has not been available so far in the literature. Our results show that similar to findings of exercise studies [6—9] and studies with Holter monitoring in patients with unstable angina [10—12], the presence of transient ischemia is a sign heralding a guarded prognosis. We do not know however whether it is the transient occurrence of ischemia itself that is damaging the heart, e.g., with repeated small emboli and small foci of necrosis of whether transient ischemia is only heralding subsequent ischemia with more severe symptoms.

Our study is observational. We did not intend to treat patients according to the results of their Holter monitoring, nor were they monitored after treatment had been instituted. In studies of patients with unstable angina pectoris the patients were all studied while undergoing medical treatment that seemed appropriate regarding the symptoms of the patients. The patients in our study were only taking short-acting nitrates during the period of Holter monitoring and were allowed to remain on beta-blockers in a constant dose if they had taken beta-blockers before. The results of our follow-up may have been changed by the treatment the patients received during their hospital stay of thereafter. This could, however, only influence the results in such a way as to diminish the differences betwee patients with and without transient ischemia. Thus, if differences in prognosis can be found between patients with and without ischemic episodes, these differences must be all the more valid. Like in other studies in patients with coronary artery disease, the effects of a diagnostic test on prognosis already become apparent to a great extent during the first years of follow-up. In a study of a longer follow-up on patients after unstable angina pectoris [17], prognosis over 30 days and two years varied in the same directions.

Conclusion

Our study shows that transient ischemia, as demonstrated on ambulatory electro-cardiographic monitoring, is a bad prognostic sign for patients with coronary artery disease. This does not necessarily imply that the treatment of such transient episodes will improve the prognosis of the patients. Future studies — which are quite difficult in design because of the great number of different choices for treatment — are necessary if a rationale for treatment of silent ischemic episodes is to be established.

References

1. v. Arnim Th, Maseri A (1987) Silent ischemia, current concepts and management. Steinkopff, Darmstadt, Springer, New York
2. v. Arnim Th, Erath A, Höfling, B, Schreiber MA (1987) Prevalence of silent ischemia in patients undergoing coronary angiography. In: Th. v. Arnim, A. Maseri (eds), Silent Ischemia, Current Concepts and Management, Steinkopff, Darmstadt, Springer, New York, p. 81—90

3. Cohn PF (1985) Silent myocardial ischemia and infarction. Dekker, New York—Basel
4. Rutishauser W, Roskamm H (1985) Silent myocardial ischemia, Springer, Berlin—Heidelberg—New York—Tokyo
4a. Hill JA, Pepine CF (1988) Silent myocardial ischemia. Ann Rev Med 39: 213—219
5. Kannel WB, Abbott RD (1984) Incidence and prognosis of unrecognized myocardial infarction. An update on the Framingham study. New Engl J Med 311: 1144—1147
6. Robb GP, Marks HH (1964) Latent coronary artery disease. Determination of its presence and severity by the exercise electrocardiogram. Am J Cardiol. 603—618
7. Giagnoni E, Secchi MB, Wu SC, Morabito A, Oltrona L, Mancarella S, Volpin N, Fossa L, Bettazzi L, Arangio G, Sachero A (1983) Prognostic value of exercise ECG testing in asymptomatic normotensive subjects. A prospective matched study. New Engl J Med 309: 1085—1089
8. Multiple Risk Factor Intervention Trial Research Group (1985) Exercise electrocardiogramm and coronary heart disease mortality in the multiple risk factor intervention trial. Am J Cardiol 55: 16—24
9. Gordon DJ, Ekelund LG, Karon JM; Probstfield JL, Rubenstein C, Sheffield T, Weissfeld L (1986) Predictive value of the exercise tolerance test for mortality in North American men: The lipid research clinics mortality follow-up study. Circulation 74: 252—261
10. Gottlieb SO, Weisfeldt ML, Ouyang P, Mellits ED, Gerstenblith G (1986) Silent ischemia as a marker for early unfavourable outcomes in patients with unstable angina. New Engl J Med 314: 1214—1219
11. Nademanee K, Intarachot V, Josephson MA, Rieders D, Mody FV, Singh VN (1987) Prognostic significance of silent myocardial ischemia in patients with unstable angina. J Am Coll Cardiol 10: 1—9
11a. Gottlieb SO (1987) Association between silent myocardial ischemia and prognosis: insensitivity of angina pectoris as a marker of coronary artery disease activity. Am J Cardio 60: 33J—38J
12. v. Arnim Th (1987) Silent ischemia in patients with coronary heart disease: prevalence and prognostic implications. Eur Heart J, 8. Suppl G: 115—118
12a. v. Arnim Th (1985) ST-Segment-Analyse im Langzeit EKG. DMW, 110: 1047—1051
13. v. Arnim Th, Erath A, Höfling B, Schreiber MA (1987) Prevalence of silent ischemia in patients undergoing coronary angiography. In: Th. v. Arnim, A. Maseri (eds), Silent Ischemia, Current Concepts and Management, Steinkopff, Darmstadt, Springer, New York, p. 81—90
14. v. Arnim Th, Höfling B, Schreiber MA (1985) Characteristics of episodes of ST elevation or ST depression during ambulatory monitoring in patients subsequently undergoing coronary angiography. Brit Heart J 54: 484—488
15. Selbman HK, Raab A (1978) SAVOD-Q: Sammel- und Auswertungssystem volldynamischer Datenbestände. Technische Berichte d. Inst. f. Med. Informationsverarbeitung, Statistik und Biomathematik, Universität München, Nr. 3
16. Dixon WJ (1985) BMDP — Statistical software manual. University of California Press, Berkly
17. Gottlieb SO, Weisfeldt ML, Ouyang P, Mellits D, Gerstenblith G (1987) Silent ischemia predicts infarction and death during 2 year follow-up of unstable angina. J Am Coll Cardiol 4: 756—769

Authors's address:
PD Dr. med. Th. v. Arnim
I. Medizinische Abteilung
Rotkreuzkrankenhaus
Nymphenburger Straße 163
8000 München, FRG

Discussion

KRUCOFF:

How did the Holter ECG perform relative to the exercise tests in these patients?

VON ARNIM:

In univariate analysis it performed worse for the prognosis but the exercise test was clearly covariate with the degree of fixed stenoses. So, when the influence of the Gensini score was taken out of the multivariate analysis then the independent prognostic influence of the positive exercise test is gone. That shows, that the exercise ECG is covariant with the degree of fixed stenosis. The result of the ST Holter monitoring just crosses the line of being independently significant at the 0.05 level. I think this is a hint, that Holter monitoring can tell us a little bit more than the exercise test in terms of disease activity.

KRUCOFF:

So you would say that Holter monitoring offered you independent and important information apart from exercise testing?

VON ARNIM:

Ambulatory monitoring offers independent information. How important that is, being just of marginal statistical significance, that depends on your set of patients and and whom you want to test. But it is independent information and from that point of view it tells you more than the exercise test. The exercise test is easier to perform, and if you are interested in screening patients to see whether to do a coronary angiogram on these patients, then you are better off with the exercise test. But if you have an angiogram and you have an exercise test and want to see what is the disease activity, then the Holter is a good thing to do.

FOX:

We did a similar prognostic study at the heart hospital and when we analyzed our data, we had a considerable problem. I mean especially people coming into hospital for coronary angiography, where you then make the decision to operate, which is one of your endpoints based on the angiogram, based on the symptoms, based on the exercise test - so your are, in fact, prejudging endpoints before the patient comes into the study. Many of these patients will have their operation fairly soon after they go into the study.

This makes it very difficult then to determine independent predictors of final endpoints, when you have actually used those predictors to make your decision to do the operation. For instance, you have a person with a three-vessel disease and a remarkably positive exercise test. You probably would have operated on that patient, because you have decided that is what you are going to do anyway.

VON ARNIM:

That is what comes out from the graphs and that is why these patients with triple-vessel disease have such a high rate of operation. That is quite clear. But I think that especially during 1982 we had just started with our Holter monitors. It was not of any great influence in the decision-making at that time.

FOX:

But the Holter is not completely independent of the exercise test. The Holter is quite closely inter-related with the exercise test and there may be slightly independent predictors. But it does make it difficult if you try to determine a prognostic variable on that basis when you prejudge some elements anyway.

APPELS:

Your strongest predictor was the Gensini score in your first equation, then you left your strongest predictor out and then the Holter monitoring became a predictor. Why did you leave the Gensini score out?

VON ARNIM:

To see what are independent predictors. That is the philosophy of the stepwise regression analysis in the Cox model that you look for all variables in step one and then remove one variable after the other and see how long you still have variables that give independent predictions.

GOHLKE:

In your multivariate analysis did you use a Holter positive, a Holter negative or did you also look at the separation into silent ischemic episodes vs symptomatic.

VON ARNIM:

Positive and negative, we took it altogether.

GOHLKE:

I think as far as prognostic importance of silent ischemia is concerned it might be worthwhile to look at this particularly, separating out silent ischemia.
If you were to include more unstable patients, then the Holter would become probably much more important. Again it will become much more important if in the Holter you include only those that have more than x numbers of episodes of a certain severity. For example, episodes with ST-segment elevation in patients with unstable angina. Then it would become probably by far the most important variable. When we try to rush analysis we forget about complexity and we pick up this and that, and then we come up with conclusions that are not necessarily those I would have expected, because, for example, I would expect, as shown in other studies, ejection fraction is very important. But if you do not include those patients in your group then ejection fraction does not become important if you select Holters that are very positive and so I think that, as usual, if we give to our diagnostic tools the proper investigation we can make good use of them.

VON ARNIM:

I could not agree more. This is a study where we have done the survey of our patients and that excluded unstable angina patients. The unstable ones were studied on the CCU and we have seen marked prognostic importance of that before.

MASERI:

Your curves of events are very steep during the first 12 months, then they flatten out and have the same slope for one-, two-, three-vessel disease. It looks even then that there is a certain instability although less instability than in the acute form of of unstable angina, when the patient presents. Those that survive that first year, have a good prognosis, if I may call it so, which is sort of independent of one-, two-, three-vessel disease.

VON ARNIM:

Absolutely, we noticed that trend although it was a little disappointing, because we said we could have done this study with a one-year follow-up and just similar results.

Silent ischemia pre and post PTCA — incidence and prognostic importance

C. Gohlke, H. Gohlke, J. Petersen, A. Früh, P. Betz, and H. Roskamm

Rehabilitationszentrum für Herz- und Kreislaufkranke Bad Krozingen, FRG

Introduction

Myocardial ischemia is markedly relieved by successful percutaneous transluminal angioplasty as documented by exercise testing [1—4]. In an earlier study we found [5, 6] that also Holter-detected myocardial ischemia was markedly improved after successful PTCA, but not completely abolished.

The reason for the persistent or newly appearing ischemic episodes detected by Holter post-PTCA is not known. It has also not been studied whether the degree of reduction in Holter-detected myocardial ischemia correlates with the completeness of revascularization achieved during PTCA. Furthermore, the prognostic significance of ischemic episodes registered post-PTCA is unknown.

Thus the goals of the present study were:
1) To determine the incidence of silent ischemic episodes pre and post PTCA in a larger number of patients;
2) To evaluate the prognostic importance of silent ischemic episodes post PTCA.

Methods

Between October, 1986 and June, 1988, 127 patients with primary successful PTCA and complete 24 h Holter monitoring pre and post PTCA were examined. PTCA was defined as primary successful if the dilated stenosis was reduced to less than 50% of luminal diameter. Excluded were patients with conduction disturbances, atrial fibrillation and marked left ventricular hypertrophy. In all patients the influence of positional changes on ST-T-segments was tested, to exclude false positive ST-depression.

All 127 patients underwent 24 h Holter-monitoring, three to eight days before and after PTCA, using the Oxford Medilog 4500 system for ST-segment registration. The following parameters were evaluated: the number of symptomatic and asymptomatic ischemic episodes, the duration of ST-segment depression in minutes, maximal ST-segement-depression in mV, and heart-rate at maximal ST-segment-depression.

An ischemic episode during ambulatory ECG-monitoring was defined as ST-segment-depression of > 0.1 mV, of > 1 minute in duration, separated from a second episode by more than 1 minute.

Pre PTCA all patients were examined under antianginal drug regimens, usually consisting of a combination of nitrates, betablockers, and calcium-antagonists; in addition, patients received acetyl-salicylic-acid in dosages between 100 and 500 mg.

During the 24 hour following PTCA patients were monitored in the coronary care unit and maintained on nitro-glycerin 3—6 mg per hour via perfusion pump until the following morning; they also received retarded nifedipine 20 mg q 8 h. After 24 h patients were returned to their regular ward and were fully ambulatory. They received retarded nifedipine 3×20 mg, isosorbide dinitrate 20 mg in the morning and at noon, as well as acetyl-salicylic-acid 500 mg. Betablockers were only given as clinically indicated for hypertension or rhythm disturbances.

Right heart catheterization during symptom limited supine bicycle ergometry was performed within one week before and after PTCA with measurement of pulmonary capillary wedge pressure, cardiac index, and ST-segment-depression at the highest work load. All medications were discontinued 12 hours before the exercise test.

Fifty patients underwent angiography using Judkins or Sones technique on the average 4.8 months after PTCA for assessment of degree of restenosis.

Hemodynamic data are presented as mean values $\pm$ SEM. Comparisons were made using a paired t-test. To determine the significance of Holter monitor-detected ischemia before versus after angioplasty a chi-square analysis was used. The significance level was set at $p < 0.05$. The duration of episodes before and after PTCA was compared using the Wilcoxon ranks test. All calculations were performed on a VAX 11/750 using the BMDP statistical software package of the University of California.

Results

The mean age of 127 patients was 54 years; 17% were female; 64% had single vessel disease, 28% had double, and 8% had triple vessel disease. In 75.4% of patients the LAD was dilated, in 15.9% the right coronary artery, the circumflex in 7.1%, and the diagonal branch in 1.6%.

The incidence of ischemic episodes during 24 h Holter monitoring pre and post PTCA is shown in Table 1. Forty-two patients (33%) had ischemic episodes, pre PTCA, 73% of those were silent. Three to eight days post-PTCA — on the average 4.5 days — ischemic episodes were registered in 27 of 127 patients (21%), 95% of those were silent. The total number of episodes was reduced by 50% from 121 episodes pre PTCA to 60 post PTCA. Silent episodes were reduced by 35% from 88 to 57 episodes and symptomatic ischemic episodes by 91% from 33 to 3 episodes.

Table 1. Incidence of ischemic episodes pre and post PTCA

	pre	post
	PTCA	
Number of patients examined	127	127
Number of patients with ischemic episodes	42 (33%)	27 (21%)
percent of silent episodes	73%	95%

The mean duration of ischemic episodes was significantly reduced from 24 ± 5 min to 14 ± 4.0 min (p < 0,01) and also the percent of episodes lasting longer than 60 min was reduced from 14 to 7%.

Pre PTCA the majority of episodes occurred between 06.00 and 12.00 hrs (42%); 29% of episodes were registered between 12.00 and 18.00 hrs; 24% between 18.00 and 24.00 hrs; and only 5% of episodes occurred between 2400 and 0600 hrs.

Post PTCA the diurnal distribution of ischemic episodes was mitigated, but still most episodes occurred between 06.00 and 12.00 hrs (38.3%), followed by 31% of episodes between 12.00 −18.00 hrs, and 24% between 1800 and 2400 hrs; 8% of episodes occurred between 24.00 and 06.00 hrs (Fig. 1).

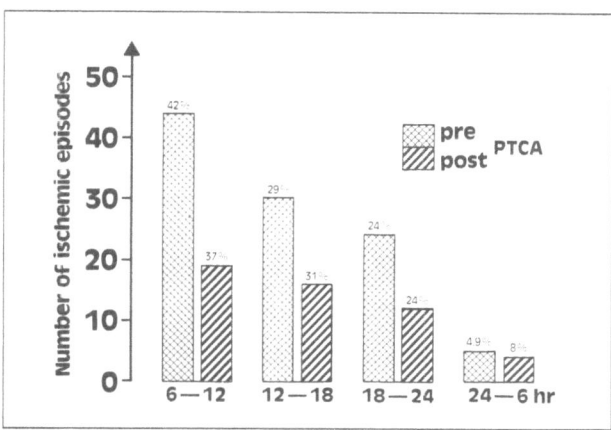

Fig. 1. Diurnal variation in incidence of ischemic episodes pre and post PTCA

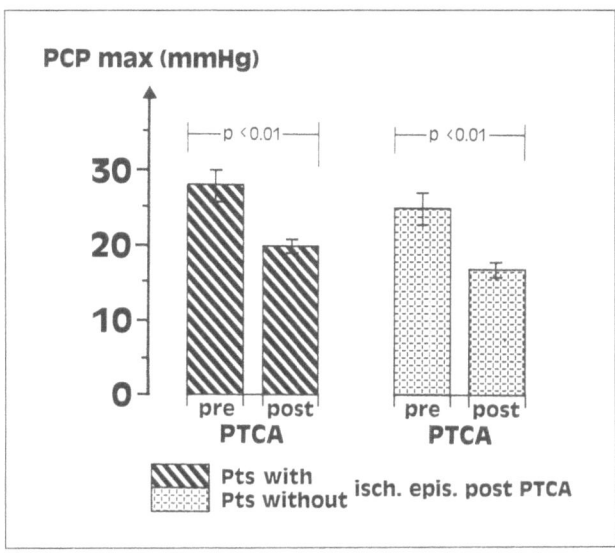

Fig. 2. Pulmonary capillary wedge pressure, mmHg during peak exercise in pts with and without ischemic episodes post PTCA

In an attempt to identify characteristics of patients with and without ischemic episodes post PTCA, we analyzed the incidence of ischemic episodes pre PTCA in those tow groups. Sixty-seven percent of 27 patients with ischemic episodes post PTCA had ischemic episodes pre PTCA in contrast to 24% of 100 patients in whom ischemic episodes were absent post PTCA ($p < 0.01$).

Eighteen of 27 patients with ischemic episodes post PTCA and 65 of 100 patients without ischemic episodes post PTCA underwent right heart catheterization during symptom-limited exercise within one week post PTCA.

Fifty-six percent of patients with ischemic episodes post PTCA had ST-segment-depression during exercise in comparison to 32% of patients without ischemic episodes post PTCA.

In order to evaluate if the presence of ischemic episodes post PTCA correlates with the hemodynamic findings during exercise, we evaluated pulmonary capillary wedge pressure and cardiac output during symptom-limited exercise in patients with and without ischemic episodes post PTCA. In spite of a significantly higher cardiac output achieved during exercise, the post PTCA pulmonary wedge pressure is significantly lower than pre PTCA. This improvement in cardiac function, is represented by the decrease in pulmonary capillary wedge pressure (30% vs 29%) (Fig. 2) and an increase in cardiac output (Fig. 3) is comparable in both groups (24% vs 16%). Also the increase in exercise tolerance post PTCA was the same in both groups (29%) (Fig. 4). These results indicate that silent ischemic episodes post PTCA are not indicative of an inadequate dilatation.

To determine if the presence of silent ischemic episodes is a risk factor for early restenosis, we reviewed the angiograms of 50 patients who had undergone coronary angiography (on the average of 4.8 months post PTCA) for recurrent symptoms or severe signs of ischemia during exercise tests. Only one patient had neither symptoms nor ischemia and was examined for occupational reasons. The incidence of silent ischemic episodes in patients with restenosis was 17% (4 of 22 patients); in patients without restenosis it was 23%.

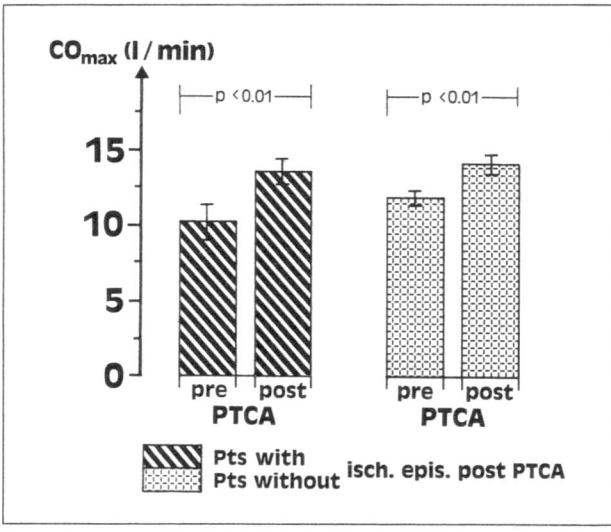

Fig. 3. Cardiac output during peak exercise (l/min) in patients with and without ischemic episodes post PTCA

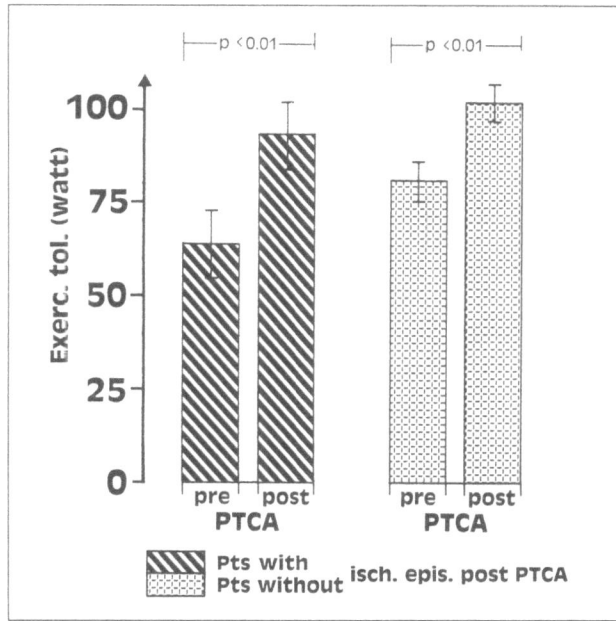

Fig. 4. Exercise tolerance (w) in patients with and without ischemic episodes post PTCA

silent ischemic episodes in patients with restenosis was 17% (4 of 22 patients); in patients without restenosis it was 23%.

Conclusions

Six months post PTCA out patient follow-up with 24-h Holter monitoring in 31 patients revealed a decrease in incidence of ischemic episodes. Although all patients were now more active only 3 of 11 patients who had ischemic episodes one week post PTCA still showed ischemic episodes after 6 months.

PTCA leads to a significant reduction in total number and duration of ischemic episodes with almost complete abolition of symptomatic episodes. Silent ischemic episodes are improved by PTCA to a lesser degree than symptomatic ischemic episodes and are still present in 21% of patients. The diurnal distribution of ischemic essentiallyepisodes shows the highest incidence between 06.00 and 12.00 hrs. This is mitigated after PTCA. Patients with silent ischemic episodes post PTCA have also a higher incidence of silent ischemic episodes pre PTCA. Functional and hemodynamic improvement is comparable in patients with and without silent ischemic episodes. Silent ischemic episodes are not indicative of an inadequate dilatation and they cannot be considered a risk factor for early restenosis.

Within 6 months post PTCA the incidence of ischemic episodes present within the first week post PTCA decreases.

The reason for the persistence of, or newly appearing silent ischemic episodes post PTCA is not known and deserves further evaluation. A possible explanation could be a traumatically induced, increased vascular tone in susceptible patients, or platelet aggregation on endothelial lesions, which may disappear with the healing process of the vessel wall.

References

1. Gruentzig AR, Senning A, Siegenthaler WE (1979) Nonoperative dilatation of coronary artery stenosis. Percutaneous transluminal coronary angioplasty. N Engl J Med 301: 61—68
2. Scholl JM, Chaitmann BR, David PR et al. (1982) Exercise electrocardiography and myocardial scintigraphy in the serial evaluation of the results of percutaneous transluminal coronary angioplasty. Circulation 66: 380—390
3. Meier B, Gruentzig AR, Siegenthaler WE, Schlumpf M (1983) Long term exercise performance after percutaneous transluminal coronary angioplasty and coronary artery bypass grafting. Circulation 68: 796—802
4. Rosing DR, Van Raden M, Mincemoyer RM, et al. (1984) Exercise, electrocardiographic and functional response after percutaneous transluminal coronary angioplasty. Am J Cardiol 53: 36C—41C
5. Gohlke C, Gondolf K, Gohlke H, Petersen J, Roskamm H (1987) Stumme Ischämie vor und nach PTCA. Z Kardiol 76: Suppl II
6. Gohlke C, Gohlke, H, Petersen J, Fruh A, Roskamm H (1988) Is silent ischemia after PTCA of prognostic importance? — a prospective study. Europ. H. J. Suppl. 1, Vol 9 p. 155

Authors address:
Dr. Christa Gohlke-Bärwolf
Rehabilitationszentrum
für Herz- und Kreislaufkranke
D-7812 Bad Krozingen, FRG

Discussion

KRUCOFF:

Of your patients, presumably all the single-vessel patients who were successfully dilated, you would term a complete revascularization. My first question would be, how many of your two- or three-vessel disease patients were completely revascularized, and were those who were not completely revascularized any of the people who had ST episodes? My second question is whether you saw in any of your ST episodes ST elevation, or were these exclusively episodes of ST depression?

GOHLKE:

Surprisingly enough, we did not see any ST-segment elevation in these 127 patients. We have extended this now even further, and we still have not come across ST-segment elevation. The patients with two- and three-vessel disease, of those there were only a few, four patients had dilatation in two vessels, and the other patients had only stenosis that were not more than 50%. So for all practical purpose we did consider them as completely revascularized.

KRUCOFF:

In the diminution of ST episodes that you show over your six-month period is a direct picture of what we see angiographically in the increase in lumen size with favorable healing. Whether it is platelets or whatever, there is clearly a healing process, and the lumen of the dilatation site increases over that six-month period, just as your ST episodes have faded away.

ANDRESEN:

If you look not only to the total patient group post and pre-PTCA but look for the individual patient, and look for whether they are responders or nonresponders, what happened to that group? Are there the same results? You told us that 20% or 22% of that patient group had ischemia post PTCA. Was it the same group as before, or do these groups differ? How many responders and nonresponders do you have?

GOHLKE:

There is a slight diversion. 15% of patients who had ischemic episodes pre-PTCA had either the same degree or an increase. And the rest of the patients were compiled of those who did not have ischemic episodes pre-PTCA, so they were patients in whom ST-segment depression occurred newly after PTCA. There was no difference between those in their reaction and in their characteristics as far as the number of vessels involved is concerned.

ANDRESEN:

How would you explain the fact that somebody has pre-PTCA no ST segment changes, but only post PTCA?

GOHLKE:

I think it may be the variability and the degree of trauma that one applies to the PTCA site. In some patients, if you look at the angios afterwards some look beautiful, and some look rather ragged. That may be an explanation for it. We are trying to get at this question by restudying these patients with quantitative angiography. But we are in the process of doing this, which is rather time-consuming and tedious.

DE CATERINA:

One of the most striking findings is the reduction in symptomatic episodes after PTCA. I wonder, did you correlate these with decreasing mean severity of episodes or mean duration of episodes after the procedure?

131

GOHLKE:

The mean duration of episodes dramatically decreases also post-PTCA. We all talk about patients who have silent ischemia, ST-segment depression, but nobody talks about those patients who have symptoms without ST-segment depression. We have looked at this too, and also that the incidence of symptomatic episodes, whether accompanied by ST-segment depression or not, decreases post-PTCA. That may be due to the placebo effect of PTCA, but I not think so. One possible explanation might be that some nerve pathways also get disturbed, and this has so far not been well examined.

KRUCOFF:

Let me add that in a completely independent experience using four different angiographic definitions of restenosis and looking at the acute ECG changes in the first 24 h of monitoring, there is no correlation with restenosis between how these lesions behave in the first 24 h and what they look and act like in the next three to six months.

APPELS:

Your explanation seems to be the traumata induced by the angioplasty itself. But could the mental status of the patients influence the silent ischemia, too?

GOHLKE:

If the mental status of these patients who have undergone PTCA is changed, I think it is only changed in a very positive way, because they are all so happy post-PTCA, they feel much better, I think that all of these negative parameters, which you showed so well yesterday, might have been present pre-PTCA but should not play a role post-PTCA.

APPELS:

In that case PTCA would be the best psychiatry in the world.

SIEGRIST:

Well it is a call for an even more interdisciplinary approach.

MASERI:

Did you try to correlate the result in individual patients of exercise testing and the result of the Holter?

GOHLKE:

Yes, we did, and there is a quite good correlation.

Acute ischemic syndromes and progression of coronary atherosclerosis

W. Rafflenbeul

Hannover Medical School, Hannover, FRG

The natural course of coronary atherosclerosis has to be studied by repeat coronary angiograms during medical treatment of patients over prolonged periods of time. Although numerous coronary angiographies are carried out each year only a limited number of patients are restudied under controlled conditions.

Furthermore, conclusions from repeated angiographic studies might be fraught with substantial pitfalls, some of which are:
1) Since most patients are selected for restudy because of persistence or progression of clinical symptoms the study population might be short on patients with stable disease and obviously excludes all patients whose disease progression had a fatal course;
2) To include patients with differing severity of coronary artery disease might be inappropriate, as will be emphasized later;
3) Because, in most instances, the second angiogram is only performed to reassess suitability for bypass surgery most studies:
   a) are designed retrospectively,
   b) show a highly variable time interval between angiograms, and
   c) are mostly poorly controlled.
4) Over prolonged intervals between coronary angiograms the x-ray-equipment might be upgraded. Technical aspects like unchanged exposure conditions, equal film quality, and film processing procedures might influence the interpretation results. In addition, consistent interpretation is dependent on matching angle and sequence of views to facilitate simultaneous reading of both angiograms. In most studies severity of the coronary artery disease is assessed by qualitative criteria which are — despite sophisticated scoring systems — too often fraught with both intra- and interobserver variability.
5) Even when quantitative measurements are taken — as we have done for several years — the physiologic state of the patient during coronary angiography may substantially influence the results. Dynamic changes in luminal diameter due to different vasomotor tone, platelet aggregation, or thrombolysis may alter the angiographic appearance of the disease.

Although it is difficult to eliminate all the bias introduced by these pitfalls completely, most follow-up studies give valuable information concerning the evolution of coronary artery disease as assessed by repeated coronary arteriography [3—10, 12—20].

With respect to the specific topic of this workshop two major interim parameters are closely related to progressive coronary artery disease:
1) the time interval between studies and
2) evolution of clinical symptoms, particularly the appearance of unstable angina.

Time interval

Despite a large overlap, most studies show a trend towards more progression with an increasing time interval. On the average, 58% of patients demonstrated progressive disease at angiography already after one to two years, 65% between three and five years, and up to 85% after more than five years. This course is confirmed by regression lines computed from large scale interval studies from individual institutions (Fig. 1): about 50% of patients had progressive coronary artery disease after two years and about 80% after five years observation period. With prolonged periods of time, alterations of coronary atheroma associated with acute ischemic syndromes are more likely to occur. Coronary arteries with advanced atherosclerotic plaques often demonstrate at post morten analysis (see Davies, M.J., this volume) fragmentation of elastic elements and enhanced softening due to fatty deposits. With such fragile atherosclerotic plaque it is more likely that already the normal bending and twisting of the coronary vessels during contraction of the heart as well as variations in vasomotor tone or changes in blood pressure result in rupture of the weak fibrous cap with subsequent thrombus formation. This "coronary accident" leads to rapid

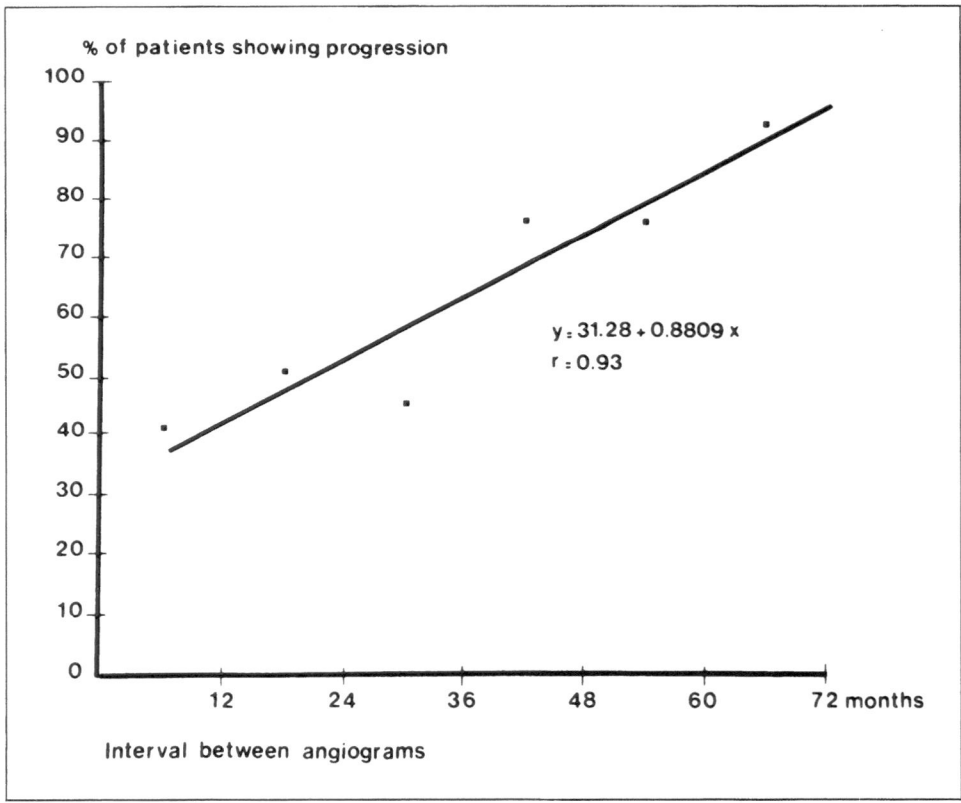

Fig. 1. The regression line represents the percentage of patients with progressive coronary artery disease in relation to the time interval between angiographic studies (reprinted from [5]).

increase of a focal arterial narrowing and is regarded as the most frequent cause of unstable angina or myocardial infarction.

Evolution of clinical symptoms

According to the pathophysiological concept of a "complicated" atherosclerotic plaque as one prerequisite for acute ischemic syndromes, worsening of exertional angina, crescendo angina, and particularly angina at rest, are often associated with progressive coronary artery disease on subsequent angiography if compared with a previous coronary angiogram.

Moise et al. [13] analyzed progression of coronary lesions in patients who had a previous angiography and were later hospitalized for an episode of unstable angina and compared it with angiographic progression of patients with stable angina who also had two interval angiograms. They found progression of a coronary stenotic segment in 76% (29 out of 38) of patients after an episode of unstable angina but only in 31% (12 out of 38) of patients with a stable clinical course. In 21 patients (= 55%) with unstable angina progression to at least a 70%, stenosis occurred, but only in five patients (= 13%) with a quiet interval. Progression in initially normal segments or multifocal progression were also more frequent in the unstable angina group of patients.

Therefore, progression in the extent and the severity of coronary obstructive lesions is commonly found in patients with a history of stable angina who have undergone repeat angiography after an episode of unstable angina.

Ambrose et al. [1] analyzed the coronary artery morphology of patients with such an acute coronary syndrome. They found the eccentric lesion with a narrow neck due to one or more overhanging edges and irregular borders (type II lesion) the most common morphologic feature. As demonstrated in Fig. 2, it was found in 12 out of

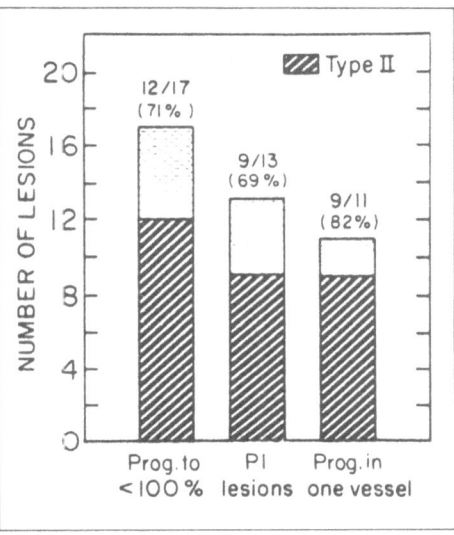

Fig. 2. Incidence and percentage of type II lesions in patients restudied after an episode of unstable angina. Prog. = progression; P.I. = previously insignificant. (Reprinted from [1]).

17 lesions that progressed to <100% in patients with unstable angina but in only 16% of patients with stable angina. Of the 13 lesions which progressed from an initially insignificant degree of obstruction, nine, i.e., 69% were of type II. And in 11 patients, who had only one stenosis progressive, nine, i.e., 82% were type II lesions. Recent post mortem angiographic and pathologic analysis (see Davies, M. J. this volume) as well as information obtained with intraoperative coronary angioscopy have confirmed that such eccentric angiographic lesions represent ruptured atherosclerotic plaques with associated thrombi.

Figure 2 demonstrates another important fact with regard to abrupt progression of coronary artery disease. Of 17 progressive coronary obstructions, 13 were only insignificant at the initial angiography. Although the degree of narrowing just before the onset of the unstable angina period is not known exactly, it is most likely that the significant obstruction at repeat angiography had not developed slowly but is the consequence of a "coronary accident" with a distruption of a moderately encroaching plaque.

This fact is further substantiated by a recent retrospective study of the same group in patients with repeat angiography after acute myocardial infarction (Fig. 3). In the patients with myocardial infarction, 11 out of 23, i.e., 48% of lesions, were initially less than 50% and only five, i.e., 22%, were more than 70%. The rapid evolution of coronary artery disease, often associated with a worsening of clinical symptoms, seems to be a random phenomenon which may occur every time during the natural course of coronary artery disease.

Based on these facts and on clinical experience we assume that basically two distinctively different types of progression exist (Table 1): primarily progression rep-

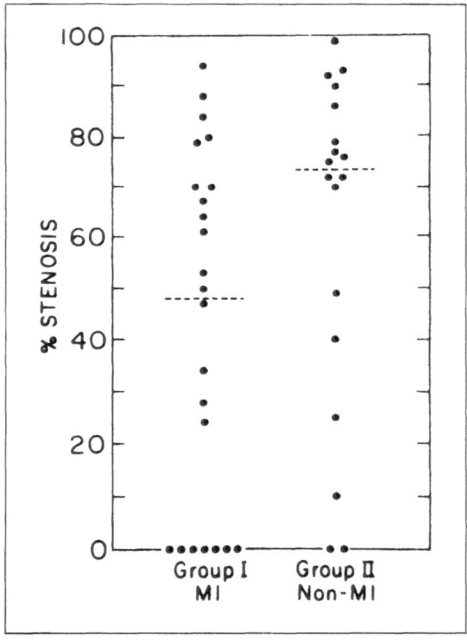

Fig. 3. Percent stenosis of infarct-related artery in the initial angiogram in 23 patients restudied after an acute myocardial infarction (group I) compared to 18 patients without interval myocardial infarction (group II). (Reprinted from [2].)

Table 1: Characteristics of primary and secondary progression of coronary artery disease (reprinted from [11]).

	Primary progression	Secondary progression
Pathophysiology	Formation or 'growth' of the atherosclerotic plaques by: ● Lipid accumulation ● Cellular proliferation ● Necrosis/fibrosis ● Calcification	Rapid enlargement of the plaque by: ● Thrombus formation ● Hemorrhage ● Vasoconstriction
Time interval	Years (with variable speed)	Minutes-hours
Clinical symptoms	Slowly progressive angina pectoris (stepwise)	Sudden deterioration of angina pectoris (unstable angina pectoris, acute myocardial infarction)

resents the formation or growth of a plaque by the basic atherosclerotic process taking place over years — possibly in bouts — and is characterized clinically by a slowly progressive exertional angina pectoris. On the other hand, secondary progression describes more rapid changes in luminal narrowing by the formation of a platelet thrombus on a distrupted atherosclerotic plaque of differing size. Intramural hemmorrhage or sudden increase of vasomotor tone may further increase the severity of obstruction and lead to unstable angina or acute myocardial infarction.

References

1. Ambrose JA, Winters SL, Rohit RA, Eng A, Riccio A, Gorlin R, Fuster V (1986) Angiographic evaluation of coronary artery morphology in unstable angina. JAAC 7/3: 472—478
2. Ambrose JA, Tannenbaum MA, Alexoupoulos D, Hjemdahl-Monsen CE, Leavy J, Weiss M, Borrico S, Gorlin R, Fuster V (1988) Angiographic progression of coronary artery disease and the development of myocardial infarction. JACC 12/1: 56
3. Bemis CE, Gorlin R, Kemp HG, Herman MV (1973) Progression of coronary artery disease: a clinical angiographic study. Circ 47: 455
4. Ben-Zvi J, Hildner PJ, Javier RP, Fester A, Samet P (1974) Progression of coronary artery disease. Cinearteriographic and clinical observations in medically and surgically treated patients. Am J Cardiol 34: 295
5. Bruschke AVG, Wijers TS, Kolsters W, Landmann J (1981) The anatomic evolution of coronary artery disease demonstrated by coronary arteriography in 256 nonoperated patients. Circ 63: 527—536
6. Frick MH, Valle M, Harjola PT (1983) Progression of coronary artery disease in randomized medical and surgical patients over a 5 year angiographic follow-up. Am J Cardiol 52: 681
7. Gensini GG, Kelly AE (1972) Incidence and progression of coronary artery disease. An angiographic correlation in 1263 patients. Arch Intern Med 129: 814
8. Kimbiris D, Lavine P, Van den Brock H, Najmi M, Likoll W (1974) Devolutionary pattern of coronary atherosclerosis in patients with angina pectoris. Coronary arteriographic studies. Am J Cardiol 33: 7
9. Kramer JR, Kitazume H, Proudfit WL, Matsuda Y, Williams GW, Sones FM Jr (1983) Progression and regression of coronary atherosclerosis. Relation to risk factors. Am Heart J 105: 134
10. Landmann J, Klosters W, Bruschke AVG (1978) Progression der obstruktiven koronaren Herzkrankheit, dargestellt anhand wiederholter Koronarangiographie. Schweiz Med. Wschr 108: 55

11. Lichtlen PR, Rafflenbeul W (1983) Progression of coronary artery disease as judged from segmental angiography. In: 2nd Münster International Arteriosclerosis Symposium. Westdeutscher Verlag, p. 101—118
12. Moccetti T, Lichtlen P, Schönbeck M, Steinbrunn W (1976) Progression of coronary artery disease based on cineangiographic data. In: Coronary angiography and angina pectoris. P. R. Lichtlen (ed), Thieme, Stuttgart, p. 88
13. Moise A, Theroux P, Toeymanges Y, Descoings B, Lesperance J, Waters DD, Pelletier GB, Bourassa MG (1983) Unstable angina and progression of coronary arteriosclerosis. N Eng J Med 309: 685—689
14. Moise A, Theroux P, Taeymans J, Waters DD, Lesperance J, Fines P, Descoings B, Robert P (1984) Clinical and angiographic factors associated with progression of coronary artery disease. JACC 3: 659—667
15. Nash DT, Gensini CG, Simon H, Arno I, Nash S (1977) The Erysichthon Syndrome. Progression of coronary atherosclerosis and dietary hyperlipidemia. Circ 56: 363
16. Palac RT, Hwang MH, Meadows WR, Croke RP, Pifarre R, Loeb HS, Gunnar RM (1981) Progression of coronary artery disease in medically and surgically treated patients 5 years after randomization. Circ 64 (Suppl. II), 17
17. Rösch J, Antonovic R, Trenouth RS, Rahimtoola SH, Sim DN, Dotter CT (1976) The natural history of coronary artery stenosis. A longitudinal angiographic assessment. Radiol 119: 513
18. Roskamm H, Stürzenhofecker P, Gornandt L, Gohlke H, Haakshorst W (1980) Progression and regression of coronary artery disease in postinfarction patients less than 40 years of age. Cleve Clin Q 47, 192
19. Shub C, Vlietstra RE, Smith HC, Fulton RE, Elveback IR (1981) The unpredictable progression of symptomatic coronary artery disease. A serial clinical angiographic analysis. Mayo Clin Proc 56: 155
20. Vanhaecke J, Piessens J, van de Werf F, Willems JL; de Geest H (1983) Angiographic evolution of coronary atherosclerosis in non-operated patients. Europ Heart J 4: 547

Author's address:
Prof. Dr. W. Rafflenbeul
Medizinische Hochschule Hannover
Abteilung Kardiologie
Konstanty-Gutschow-Str. 8
3000 Hannover 61, FRG

Discussion

HÖFLING:

Certainly angiography is a very good method to visualize a vessel and to visualize a stenosis but it is a critical method to further differentiate the stenosis. Do you think that newer technologies such as digital subtraction angios help to give a further differentiation of stenoses?

RAFFLENBEUL:

With regard to stenosis severity that might be; there are only few data on this promising method and I think we cannot conclude at this time that the digital subtraction angiography will be really an improvement. I think the most important step is to go from sight guessing to quantitative analysis and to keep the physiological state of the patient as identical as possible.

DAVIES:

I would very much agree with the distinction between primary progression and secondary progression. I think we can take it a little further and say the primary progression is really smooth muscle proliferation and has less to do with lipid and thrombus than secondary progression. I think one element of hope is that when you discover how to control smooth muscle proliferation after angioplasty you may have learned something about how to prevent primary progression of atheroma as well.

An important conceptual point is that one element of atheroma which may be a rather separate element is smooth muscle proliferation, one day perhaps we should be able to control that.

FOX:

I think that the point you made is one of the problems that we certainly have, that in people developing acute myocardial infarction the secondary lesions are often because of rather minor atheromatous narrowing, and, of course, this is one of the big problems that we have when we are using things like silent ischemia to predict which people are going to undergo infarction. If I can put a question to you and perhaps to Mike Davies: Is it correct that in a very large proportion of patients undergoing acute infarction the site of infarction is a minor narrowing not a severe narrowing, which is the one that usually causes our excitement when we look at an angiogram?

RAFFLENBEUL:

It is about 50% in this particular study, it was a similar amount in the Hammersmith study, and I have seen the data just in Rome at the atherosclerosis meeting from the stroke people and they had a similar amount of minor lesions in the carotid arteries. So, from an angiographic point of view, this is a very important point and it is unclear if we should have, for example, PTA on these minor lesions.

DAVIES:

I do wish those of you who do angiography would stop thinking that you had any knowledge of the size of a plaque. You have knowledge of how much it is causing obstruction, you have no knowledge of its size at all, and an awful lot of the plaques may well be bulging outwards and some of those plaques are very dangerous for future events. I well remember, Kim, speaking to the Cardiac Society about eight years ago and making the point that plaques that were not causing stenosis could be dangerous, and now you have discovered it yourself.

FOX:

I am getting concerned, Mike, the plaques causing stenosis are less dangerous than the ones not causing stenosis, and that really is a problem for us.

DAVIES:

I think many of the plaques that are causing high-grade stenosis are what we rightly have heard described as primary progression. They are the smooth muscle fibrous proliferating plaques, which may cause chronic high-grade stable stenosis, but they do not have as high a risk of the acute event.

The pathology of the unstable ischemic syndromes

M. J. Davies

British Heart Foundation Cardiovascular Pathology Unit, St. George's Hospital Medical School, London, UK

Conclusion

Both alterations in vasomotor tone and coronary thrombi acting in isolation or together can cause acute ischemic syndromes. Vasomotor tone variation occurs when atheromatous plaques are situated eccentrically leaving an arc of normal vassel wall. Enhanced vasoconstriction at such lesions may reflect endothelial dysfunction and/or deposition of a monolayer of platelets. Larger thrombi, detectable angiographically, are a reflection of either superficial or deep intimal injury due to atheroma. In superficial injury the endothelium is lost of points of high grade stenosis and where there is intense infiltration of the intima with lipid-filled macrophages. Deep intimal injury is due to tears extending from the lumen into the interior of plaques filled with free cholesterol. Such plaque fissures allow both an intraintimal and intraluminal thrombus to form.

Basic pathology of atherosclerosis

The basic process of atherosclerosis is a slowly progressive intimal thickening in focal areas of the arterial wall. The intima is thickened by a combination of smooth muscle proliferation, deposition of connective tissue matrix proteins including collagens together with the accumulation of a varying amount of lipid. The focal and proliferative nature of the disease is expressed in the formation of localized segments of arterial obstruction. The basic process is regarded as slowly progressive and thought to be initiated very early in life, even so the clinical course in many patients is characterized by acute episodes and the growth of plaques, as observed in sequential angiograms, is phasic [54].

Structure of stenoses due to atherosclerosis

High grade stenoses show a considerable range of morphological expression. Plaques may be concentric, that is, involve the whole circumference of the intima, or be eccentric involving only one segment of the intima (Fig. 1). The medial muscle behind intimal thickening due to atherosclerosis atrophies, thus concentric lesions do not allow any variation in the cross-sectional area of the lumen, in contrast

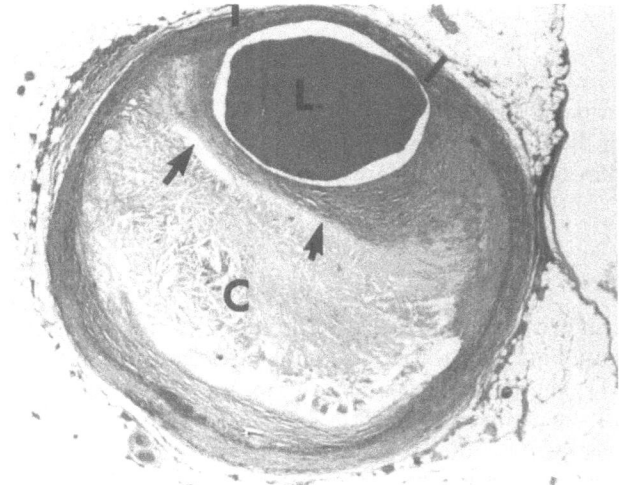

Fig. 1. Histological cross section of an eccentric coronary artery plaque. The lumen (L) contains, but is not quite filled by, angiographic medium. The plaque contains a clear zone within the intima containing cholesterol (C). This cholesterol is separated from the lumen by a thin cap fo fibrous tissue (arrows). Opposite the plaque between the two marked lines is a normal sement of arterial wall.

eccentric plaques allow retention of an arc of normal vessel wall around part of the lumen and there is the potential for tonal variation in lumen size. The plaques also vary in the relative proportions of connective tissue and lipid they contain. Hard plaques consist almost entirely of collagen; in contrast soft plaques contain a large pool of cholesterol and its esters. Such soft plaques have a potential space within the connective tissue of the intima within which lipid is incarcerated. The lipid within the pool is separated from the lumen by a cap of fibrous (Fig. 1).

Endothelial structure over normal and atherosclerotic intima

The intima contains abundant collagen, a potent platelet adhesion agonist via the platelet surface receptor. Contact between platelets and collagen is prevented by the intact endothelium in the normal vessel. Experimental denudation of the endothelium via mechanical trauma or air drying or thermal injury will invoke arterial thrombosis. In such models [6, 7, 31] the relation between the depth of intimal injury and flow or shear rates in the vessel has given valuable insights into human thrombosis. Superficial injury at low shear rates results in a single layer of platelets only, deep injury exposes the more potent type I and III collagens in larger areas, and at high shear rates this may allow larger thrombi to develop.

The question arises inevitably as to whether endothelial integrity is lost in human atherosclerotic arteries. In animal models of atherosclerosis [23, 50] fully developed plaques do show loss of endothelium with platelet adhesion as a monolayer. It should be stressed that this is neither observed in the initial phase of plaque development nor causes thrombosis of the magnitude to be recognized by angiography. Evidence is accumulating in man that endothelial function and integrity is altered in an identical manner over established plaques.

141

Pathology of unstable ischemic syndromes in man

Two possible mechanisms, thrombosis and alterations in vasomotor tone, exist for sudden local alterations in coronary flow within one epicardial artery. While evidence for the existence of both these mechanisms will be reviewed it is likely that neither exists commonly in isolation and the two are combined in many patients.

Coronary thrombosis

In patients who present suddenly with acute regional infarction and the crescendo form of unstable angina the acute nature of the event is linked to thrombosis in or on an atherosclerotic plaque [31]. The same is true of approximately 70% of subjects who die suddenly from ischemic heart disease [19, 56]. The underlying thrombotic state is so well established by necropsy studies [18, 24, 37, 48] and angiography [1, 2, 3, 4, 5, 21, 31, 32, 42, 55, 60], or angioscopy in life [28, 52] that it will not be reviewed here. What will be reviewed are the processes within the arterial wall which invoke thrombosis. Reconstruction of the artery from serial histological sections shows that thrombi large enough to be detected angiographically and thus to have caused clinical symptoms have underlying intimal damage. This damage, due to atheroma, involves loss of the endothelium and exposure of collagen and occurs either as a deep or a superficial type of injury (Table I).

Thrombosis and deep intimal injury

Tears extending deep into the intima from the lumen are responsible for about 70% of major coronary thrombi. The type of plaque involved contains a pool of free extracellular cholesterol within the intima, and it is into this pool that the tear extends. The tears in the cap range in size from a crack or fissure up to a defect several millimeters across and allow blood to enter the lipid pool from the lumen [12, 19]. The result is the formation of a mass of intraintimal thrombus which will both expand the plaque and alter its configuration. Detailed examination of the whole coronary artery tree in control subjects who have coronary atheroma, but have died of other diseases [16], shows that evidence of a recent plaque fissure can be found in approximately 10% of cases. This frequency is greater in subjects with diabetes

Table 1. Contrasting Features of Superficial and Deep Intimal Injury causing Thrombosis within the Lumen.

	Superficial	Deep
Intimal Tear	absent	present
Intraintimal Thrombus	absent	present
Cholesterol Extrusion	absent	may occur
Previous Stenosis	usual	not always
Size of Artery	often smaller arteries	larger main arteries

or hypertension who have more coronary plaques. Many plaque fissures therefore probably reseal leaving the plaque larger by virtue of containing a mass of thrombus within itself. Thus plaque fissuring is an important mechanism for intermittent plaque growth.

A proportion of plaque fissures will procede however to the formation of additional thrombus within the arterial lumen and invoke clinical symptoms [19]. The thrombus forms initially as a localized mass over the site of intimal tearing and projects into, but does not occlude the lumen. The angiographic appearances of such a fissured plaque with overlying mural thrombus are characteristic (Fig. 2) and were first recognized at necropsy [19, 40]. The association of stenosis with ragged or overhanging edges and an intraluminal-filling defect became recognized as type II lesions in angiograms in life and indicated that plaque fissures with overlying mural non-occlusive thrombus could be found in many cases of unstable angina [4, 5] in

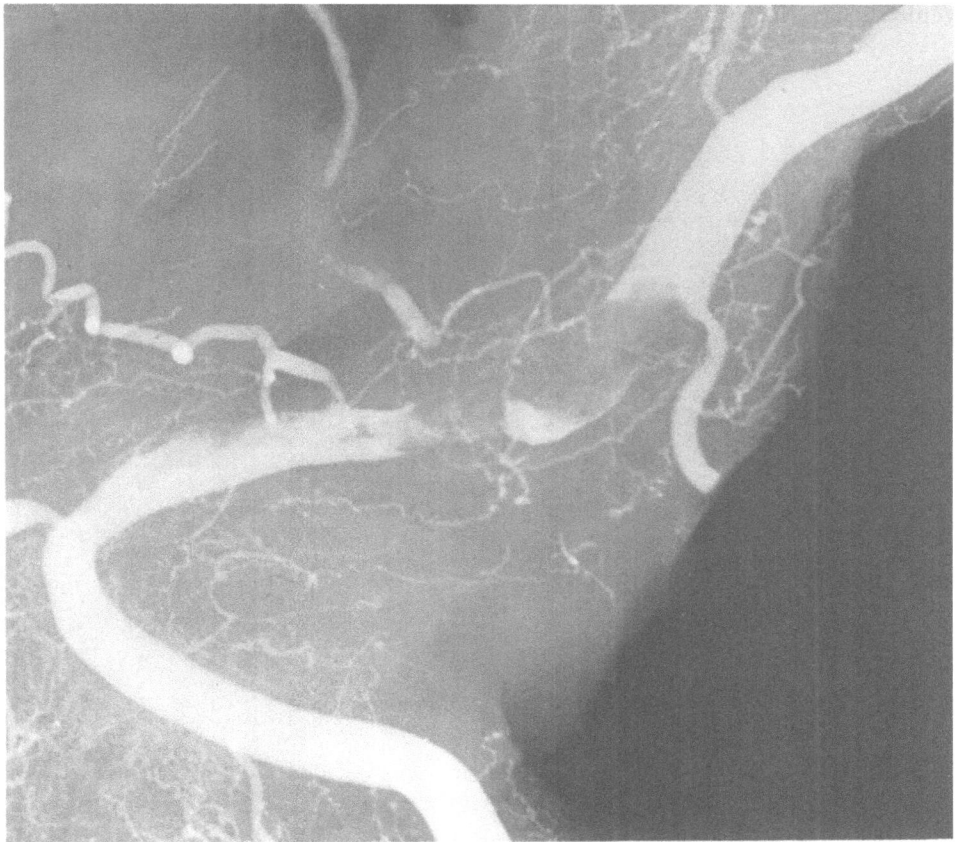

Fig. 2. Post mortem angiographic appearance of a fissured plaque with overlying mural thrombobis, but ther is still antegrade filling of the more distal coronary vessel.

143

non-transmural regional infarction [1], in arteries reopened after occlusion by fibrinolysis [3, 10], and in subjects resuscitated from out-of-hospital cardiac arrest due to ischemic heart disease [42]. Angioscopy has also confirmed the presence of mural thrombus and fissured plaques in subjects with unstable angina [28, 52].

Autopsy studies [20, 25] have shown that mural intraluminal thrombi over plaque fissures are associated with small emboli into the distal myocardium. These emboli are composed predominantly of platelets, although in some cases there is also crystalline cholesterol washed out from the plaque itself. Such emboli are associated with small microscopic foci of myocardial necrosis in the territory supplied by the artery in which the fissured plaque is situated. Autopsy studies of arteries which are completely occluded by thrombus, and associated usually with transmural regional infarction, show the ultimate development of plaque fissuring. The lumen becomes occluded by a mass of thrombus which is in continuity throughout the torn plaque cap and there is mass of thrombus within the intima (Fig. 3). Progression to the formation of an occlusive thrombus is therefore in three stages. The first is the formation of an intraintimal thrombus made up almost entirely of platelets with only a small fibrin component. Progression to the second stage, the formation of a mural intraluminal thrombus, depends upon the creation of an intensely thrombogenic surface in the fissure itself. This surface is in part exposed collagen in part a

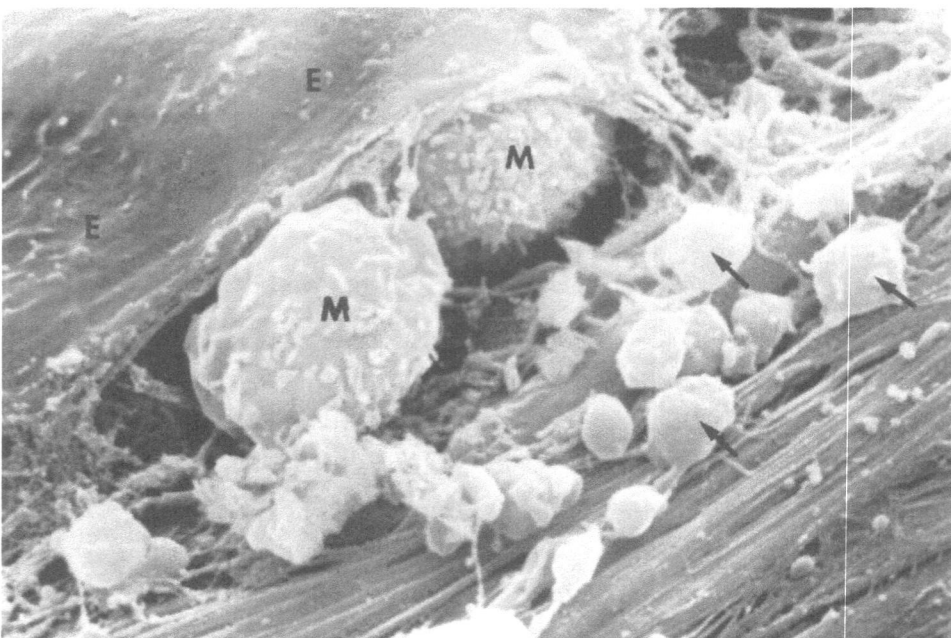

Fig. 3. Histological appearance of a large, almost occluding, intraluminal thrombus. The thrombus (black) alsmost fills the lumen and is in continuity with thrombus inside a plaque (P). The edge of the torn cap is arrowed.

layer of activated platelets. The mural thrombus has large components of both platelets and fibrin. The final third stage of occluding thrombus, and in particular the element that often propagates distally into more normal segments of artery, is predominantly composed of fibrin and red cells with a small component only of platelets. The bulk of the intraluminal thrombus is often made up of this propagation type which may well progress after the inception of infarction. Studies in which radiolabelled fibrinogen or platelets are given after myocardial infarction do show incorporation into the occluding thrombus [22, 36] but the studies of Fulton [30] show that this is in the distal tail of the thrombus, not in the proximal nidus over the fissure itself.

The sequence of events, plaque fissuring, intraintimal thrombus, mural intraluminal and occlusive thrombus must be seen as a dynamic process which can be stopped at any point and reversed. Plaque fissuring is stimulus for thrombosis formation within the lumen — whether thrombosis does occur depends on many factors, some of which are known, some speculatory.

The strength of the stimulus varies with the magnitude of the tear; some fissures allow cholesterol to be extruded and an intimal flap to be raised; occlusive thrombus is probably inevitable in such cases. Low flow and high shear rates over the lesion favor intraluminal thrombosis and are associated with either high grade preexisting stenosis, or a plaque which has rapidly grown due to the intraintimal thrombotic component. Local spasm is another factor which may reduce flow. Finally the thrombotic or fibrinolytic state at the time may influence the outcome. Plaques which fissure to cause overlying thrombosis have not necessarily caused previous high grade stenosis.

The bulk of the intraluminal thrombus, being rich in fibrin, is susceptible to lysis. Spontaneous fibrinolysis is responsible for the restoration in flow with time, observed by DeWood in his classic study of acute myocardial infarction [21]. Therapeutic fibrinolysis is equally successful in restoring flow but in both cases the underlying fissured plaque remains. Such fissured plaques heal by smooth muscle proliferation over the next few weeks and considerably remodelling of the configuration of the plaque may occur as seen in sequential angiograms. The whole process of plaque fissuring is closely analogous to the intimal injury induced by angioplasty, and the factors which control whether rethrombosis occurs and the healing process are very similar in both [14].

The time sequence of the events that lead from a plaque fissure to an occluding thrombus can only be judged from clinical data. Most subjects with the crescendo form of unstable angina will either develop acute infarction or resolve within two weeks. The former have probably progressed to complete thrombotic occlusion, the latter lysed any mural thrombus and resealed the culprit plaque fissure. In the prodromal phase of acute infarction arterial occlusion can be shown to be intermittent in many cases with waxing and waning of the thrombus within the lumen before final persistent occlusion occurs [33, 45]. The clinical impression must be that the whole sequence of plaque fissuring, thrombosis, and healing takes place over one to two weeks. There is no conclusive evidence that large areas of exposed thrombus persist in the coronary arteries at sites of plaque fissuring to provide a source of distal emboli over months in a manner analogous to ulcerated atherosclerotic plaques in the carotid arteries.

Pathogenesis of plaque fissuring

The phenomenon of plaque hemorrhage, that is the accumulation of red cells only within an atherosclerotic plaque, can be traced to bleeding from a very rich plexus of capillaries which develop in the media and cross into the thickened intima in atherosclerotic arteries [8]. Small intraplaque hemorrhage are very common but large accumulations of red cells expanding the plaque are very rare.

It is the experience of morphologists who reconstruct the microanatomy of coronary thrombi that large accumulations of platelets within the plaque can always be traced to a break in the cap with entry of blood into the intima from the arterial lumen itself.

Reconstruction of the microanatomy at autopsy of large numbers of plaques which have undergone fissuring to cause thrombi shows the vast majority are of the lipid-rich type and contain a pool of cholesterol. In most cases the lipid pool does not occupy the whole circumference of the vessel wall and the plaque cap has torn away from the adjacent more normal intima. A further characteristic of fissured plaques is the absence of internal cross struts of collagen within the pool; the implication is that there is an assymetric area of soft deformable tissue within the intima. Case reports have linked the sudden onset of coronary thrombosis with plaque rupture on exercise [9, 15].

Computer modeling of the stress patterns across plaques of this configuration do show that there are very abnormal load distributions with high stress concentrations imposed on the plaque cap. The plaque caps themselves are often thin and weak when compared to adjacent intima in mechanical tests. This structural weakness may be a reflection of the collagen being arranged is an open network packed with lipid-filled foam cells of macrophage origin which may themselves be degrading the connective tissue matrix.

Plaque fissuring is thus determined by the configuration and structure of the plaque itself, facts which do not seem susceptible to therapeutic intervention other than either preventing the formation of lipid-rich plaques or reducing the risk of thrombosis following the stimulus of a plaque fissure.

Thrombosis and superficial intimal injury

A significant minority of approximately 25% of large mural and occlusive thrombi are not due to plaque fissuring but to more superficial intimal injury at points of high grade stenosis. In some instances the intima is thickened by fibrous tissue alone, but in many there is a diffuse infiltrate of lipid-filled macrophages in the superficial layers of the intima. Thrombosis occurs over the intima in areas where the endothelial layer has apparently been lost. In this form of superficial injury there is no component of thrombus deep in the intima itself and pools of extracellular lipid are not present. Ample experimental work in atheroma induced in animals by high-lipid diets shows that heavy infiltration of the intima by macrophages containing lipid does lead to focal endothelial loss and the deposition of thin layers of platelets [23, 50]. The concordance of endothelial loss with high-grade stenosis probably accounts for thrombus formation being more pronounced in man. High-grade stenosis itself may also promote endothelial damage leading to local thrombosis [26, 59].

Vasospasm and atherosclerosis

Coronary artery spasm has been established as the basis of variant angina of the Prinzmetal type but there is also a strong association with atheroma [46, 49]. More than 50% of patients either have an irregular vessel or segments of fixed stenosis on angiography. The spasm occurs at particular sites suggesting that local reasons exist for an enhanced vasoconstrictor state.

When the intima is involved by advanced atheroma two factors prevent tonal variations in vessel lumen size. The first is the splinting effect of intimal fibrosis and calcification, while the second is the atrophy of medial smooth muscle that occurs when intimal thickness is increased by atherosclerosis. Thus many stenoses are fixed in the degree of obstruction caused. Opposite eccentric plaques, however, there is an arc of normal vessel wall remaining around part of the residual lumen [51, 58]. Clinical angiography confirms that such eccentric stenoses can be altered by vasoconstrictor and vasodilator drugs [41]. On a theorectic basis it has been argued that there is a critical relation between the length of the arc of normal media and lumen size which would allow normal tonal variation to significantly reduce flow across the lesion without having to implicate spasm. This has been put at a fixed diameter stenosis of 50% with a 60° arc of normal vessel wall [10, 11]. Up to 70% of high-grade stenoses in man have ben reported to be due to eccentric plaques and thus have a potential for variation [29].

One autopsy study of 54 males who had angina in life [34] showed 56% to have at least one high-grade eccentric stenosis. Three patients had all of their high-grade lesions of the eccentric type. Even the 44% of patients with all their lesions over 50% diameter stenosis concentric in type had eccentric lesions with lesser degree of fixed obstruction close by.

Undoubted examples of the sudden onset of unstable angina with pain at rest which can be ascribed to spasm at the site of a high grade eccentric stenosis are described [10, 11]. In one such case the variant angina persisted for two years and was due to a 56% diameter stenosis in the right coronary artery which could be varied in degree by epinephrine and nitroglycerine. Excision of this plaque at the time of insertion of coronary bybass vein graft confirmed that an arc of normal vessel wall was present.

It therefore seems that some eccentric lesions can become particularly liable to tonal variations. The reasons why a particular atherosclerotic lesion imposes an altered tone response has been the subject of intense speculation. One theory postulates there is an abnormality of the neurotransmitters which diffuse into the media from small nerves in the adventitia. An increase in lymphocytes and plasma cells as well as mast cells has been noted in the adventitia in segments of artery responsible for inducing unstable angina [27, 38]. The alternative, and perhaps more tenable view sees altered vasomotor tone as an expression of endothelial dysfunction or endothelial injury which allows the deposition of a monolayer of platelets [39, 57]. Such a monolayer would be quite impossible to detect by angiography in life.

There is a considerable body of indirect evidence that vasomotor tone abnormalities, atheroma, and platelet monolayers go together [57]. In both human and experimental atheroma the response of affected arteries is abnormal in response to the cold pressor test [47] and to the challenge of acetylcholine infusion. Acetylcholine, which is normally a vasodilator by virtue of releasing endothelial derived relaxant factor, becomes a paradoxical vasoconstrictor [13, 35, 43]. In experimental models in which the endothelium is denuded the degree of local vasoconstriction can be correlated with the number of platelets which are deposited [39]. In such areas of endothelial damage the local vasomotor responses remain abnormal for long periods suggesting that control of tone by regenerated endothelium is impaired [53]. In man it is now apparent that the endothelium over many plaques, not necessarily just those causing significant stenosis, is very abnormal [17]. There is widespread adhesion and emigration of white cells through areas of intact endothelium. Adjacent to these areas of intact endothelium is denudation injury ranging from loss of single endothelial cells to larger areas of damage exposing subendothelial matrix. Platelet adhesion in these areas is common, but as a monolayer only, and fibrin is not present (Fig. 4). Endothelial damage of this degree is closely correlated with infiltration of the intima by macrophages and some appear to be within breaches in the endothelial surface (Fig. 4). In many areas the endothelial surface is fenestrated to a degree that allows free ingress of plasma into the intima. It must be again emphasized that this endothelial damage and platelet deposition is on far too microscopic a scale for angiographic detection.

The damaged endothelial surface may have a reduced capacity for EDRF synthesis, the free access of plasma may neutralize EDRF, or platelet-derived vasoconstrictors may have free access to medial smooth muscle.

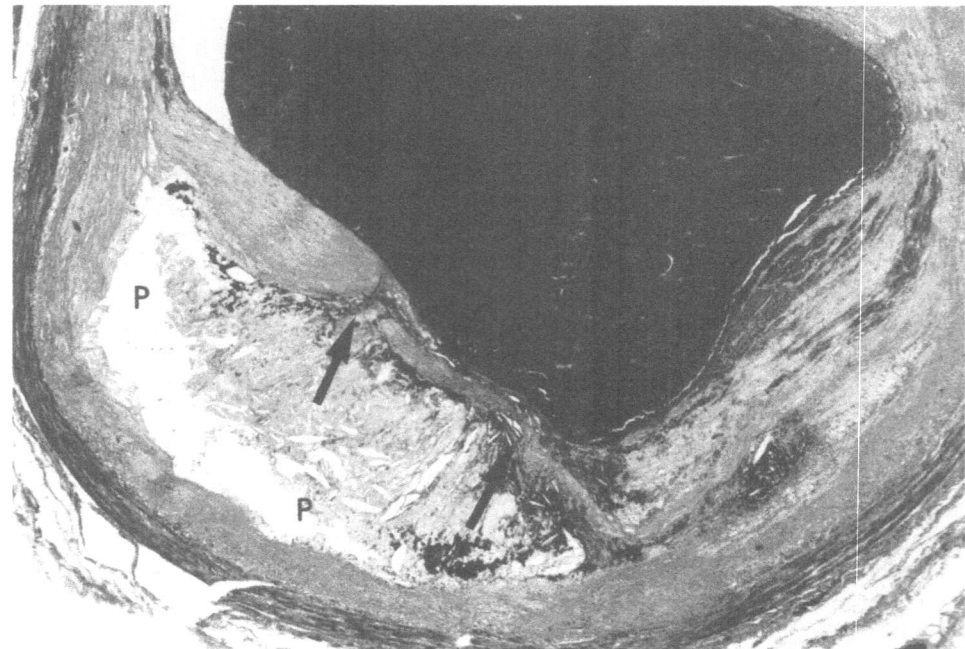

Fig. 4. Scanning electron micrograph of a human coronary artery. There is an intact endothelial cell in one area (E). In an adjacent area of denudation in jury two macrophages (M) are seen immediately beneath the endothelial surface. On the exposed subendothelial matrix platelets (arrows) are adherent.

148

Implications for clinical management

The unstable clinical syndromes of ischemic heart disease involve thrombosis and variation in vasomotor tone either acting independently or in concert. It is difficult clinically to decide the relative contribution played by each component in any individual patient at any one moment in time.

Coronary angiography will detect thrombosis when it is of a major degree and sufficient to either produce an intraluminal filling defect or occlude the lumen. The more sudden the onset and the more severe the symptoms the more likely is thrombosis to be the major component. Even so, an element of local spasm can be shown [33, 44, 45]. The longer that symptoms persist and the milder their form the more likely is for spasm to be the major component, but the possible role of platelets will be overlooked due to the insensitivity of angiography. In practice the mechanism are often determined clinically by the relative efficacy of the therapeutic drugs used in relieving the symptoms.

References

1. Ambrose JA, Hjemdahl-Monsen CE, Borrico S, Gorlin R, Fuster V (1988) Angiographic demonstration of a common link between unstable angina pectoris and non-Q-Q wave acute myocardial infarction. Am J Cardiol 61: 244—247
2. Ambrose JA, Tannenbaum MA, Alexopoulos D, Hjemdahl-Monsen CE, Leavy J, Weiss M, Borrico S, Gorlin R, Fuster V (1988) Angiographic progression of coronary artery disease and the development of myocardial infarction. JACC 12: 56—62
3. Ambrose JA, Winters SL, Arora RR et al (1985) Coronary angiograph morphology in acute myocardial infarction: link between the pathogenesis of unstable angina and myocardial infarction. J Am Coll Cardiol 6: 1233—1238
4. Ambrose JA, Winters SL, Stern A (1986) Angiographic evolution of coronary artery morphology in unstable angina. J. Am Coll Cardiol 7: 472—478
5. Ambrose JA, Winters SL, Stern A, Eng A, Teicholg LE, Gorlin R, Fuster V (1985) Angiographic morphology and the pathogenesis of unstable angina pectoris. J Am Coll Cardiol 5: 609—619
6. Badimon L, Turitto VT, Rosemark JA, Badimon JJ, Fuster V (1987) Characterization of a tubular flow chamber for studying platelet interaction with biologic and prosthetic materials: deposition of Indium-III labelled platelets on collagen, subendothelium and expanded polytetrafluoroethylene. J Lab Clin Med 110: 705—718
7. Badimon L, Badimon JJ, Galvez A, Chesebro JH, Fuster V (1986) Influence of arterial wall damage and wall shear rate on platelet deposition: Ex vivo study in a swine model. Arteriosclerosis 6: 312—320
8. Barger AC, Beeuwkes R, Lainey LL, Silverman KJ (1983) Hypothesis: vasa vasorum and neovascularisation of human coronary arteries. A possible role in the pathophysiology of atherosclerosis. New Engl J Med 310: 175—177
9. Black A, Black MM, Gensini G (1975) Exertion and acute coronary artery injury. Angiology 26: 759—783
10. Brown BG (1981) Coronary vasospasm: observations linking the clinical spectrum of ischemic heart disease to the dynamic pathology of coronary atherosclerosis. Arch Intern Med 141: 716—722
11. Brown BG, Bolson EL, Dodge HT (1984) Dynamic mechanisms in human coronary stenosis. Circulation 70: 917—922
12. Chandler AB (1974) Mechanism and frequency of thrombosis in the coronary circulation. Thromb Res 4: 3—23
13. Chappel SP, Lewis MJ, Henderson AG (1987) Effect of lipid feeding on endothelium dependent relaxation in rabbit aortic preparations. Cardiovas Res 21: 34—38
14. Chesebro JH, Lam JYT, Badimon L, Fuster V (1987) Restenosis after arterial angioplasty: a hemorrheologic response to injury. Am J Cardiol 60: 10B—16B

15. Ciampricotti R, Elgamal M (1986) Exercise induced plaque rupture producing myocardial infarction. Int J Cardiol 12: 102—108
16. Davies MJ, Bland JM, Hangartner JRW, Angelini A, Thomas AC (1989) Factors influencing the presence or absence of acute coronary thrombi in sudden ischemic death. Europ Heart J In Press
17. Davies MJ, Pepper J, Woolf N, Rowles P (1988) Endothelial integrity in human coronary arteries. Br Heart J 59: 101—101
18. Davies MJ, Thomas A (1981) The pathological basis and microanatomy of occlusive thrombus formation in human coronary arteries. Philosophical Transactions of the Royal Society of London (Biological) 294: 225—229
19. Davies MJ, Thomas AC (1985) Plaque fissuring — the cause of acute myocardial infarction, sudden ischemic death and crescendo angina. Br Heart J 53: 363—373
20. Davies MJ, Thomas AC, Knapman PA, Hangartner R (1986) Intramyocardial platelet aggregation in patients with unstable angina suffering sudden ischemic death. Circulation 73: 418—427
21. DeWood MA, Spores J, Notske R et al (1980) Prevalence of total coronary occlusion during the early hours of transmural myocardial infarction. New Engl J Med 303: 897—902
22. Erhardt LR, Unge G, Bowman G (1976) Formation of coronary arterial thrombi in relation to onset of necrosis in acute myocardial infarction in man. Am Heart J 1: 592—598
23. Faggiotto A, Ross R (1984) Studies of hypercholesterolemia in the non-human primate. II Fatty streak conversion to fibrous plaque. Arteriosclerosis 4: 341—356
24. Falk E (1983) Plaque rupture with severe pre-existing stenosis precipitating coronary thrombosis. Characteristics of coronary atherosclerotic plaques underlying fatal occlusive thrombi. Br Heart J 50: 127—134
25. Falk E (1985) Unstable angina with fatal outcome: dynamic coronary thrombosis leading to infarction and/or sudden death. Circulation 71: 699—708
26. Folts JD, Gallagher K, Rowe GG (1982) Blood flow reductions in stenosed canine coronary arteries: vasospasm or platelet aggregation. Circulation 65: 248—255
27. Forman MB, Oates JA, Robertson D et al (1985) Increased adventitial mast cells in a patient with coronary spasm. New Engl J Med 313: 1138—1141
28. Forrester JS, Litvak F, Grundfest W, Hickey A (1987) A perspective of coronary disease seen through the arteries of a living man. Circulation 75: 505—513
29. Freudenberg H, Lichtlen PR (1981) Das normale Wandsegment bei Koronartstenon, eine post mortale studie. Z Kardiol 70: 863—869
30. Fulton WFM, Sumner DJ (1976) I$_{125}$ labelled fibrinogen, autoradiography and stero-arteriography in identification of coronary thrombotic occlusion in fatal myocardial infarction. Br Heart J 38: 880—880
31. Fuster V, Badimon L, Cohen M, Ambrose JA, Badimon JJ, Chesebro J (1988) Insight into the pathogenesis of acute ischemic syndromes. Circulation 77: 1213—1220
32. Fuster V, Frye RL, Connolly DC, Danielson MA, Elveback LR, Kurland LT (1975) Angiographic patterns early in the onset of coronary syndromes. Br Heart J 37: 1250—1255
33. Hackett D, Davies G, Chierchia S, Maseri A (1987) Intermittent coronary occlusion in acute myocardial infarction: value of combined thrombolytic and vasodilator therapy. New Engl J Med 317: 1055—1059
34. Hangartner JRW, Charleston AJ, Davies MJ, Thomas AC (1986) Morphological characteristics of clinically significant coronary artery stenosis in stable angina. Br Heart J 56: 501—508
35. Heistad DD, Armstrong ML, Marcul ML, Piegors DJ, Mark AL (1984) Augmented responses to vasoconstrictor stimuli in hypercholesterolaemic and atherosclerotic monkeys. Cir Res 54: 711—718
36. Henriksson P, Edhag O, Jansson B et al (1985) A role for platelets in the process of infarct extension. New Engl J Med 313: 1660—1661
37. Horie T, Sekiguchi M, Hirosawam K (1978) Coronary thrombosis in pathogenesis of acute myocardial infarction. Histopathological study of coronary arteries in 108 necropsied cases. Br Heart J 40: 153—161
38. Kohchi K, Takebayashi S, Hiroki T, Nobuyoshi M (1985) Significance of adventitial inflammation of the coronary artery in patients with unstable angina; results at autopsy. Circulation 71: 709—716
39. Lam JYT, Chesebro JH, Steele PM, Badimon L, Fuster V (1987) Is vasospasm related to platelet deposition? Relationship in a porcine preparation of arterial injury in vivo. Circulation 75: 243—248

40. Levin DC, Fallon JT (1982) Significance of the angiographic morphology of localised coronary stenoses: Histopathological correlations. Circulation 66: 316—320
41. Lichtlen PR, Rafflenbeul WM, Freudenberg H (1985) Pathoanatomy and function of coronary obstructions leading to unstable angina pectoris; anatomical and angiographic studies. In Hugenholz PG, Goldman BS eds. Unstable Angina, Stuttgart Schattauer 81—93
42. Lo Ying-Sui A, Cutler JE, Blake K, Wright AM, Kron J, Swerdlow CD (1988) Angiographic coronary morphology in survivors of cardiac arrest. Am Heart J 115: 781—785
43. Ludmer PL, Selwyn AP, Shook TL, Wayne RR, Mudge GM, Alexander RW, Ganz P (1986) Paradoxical vasoconstriction induced by acetylcholine in atherosclerotic coronary arteries. New Engl J Med 315: 1046—1051
44. Maseri A (1987) Role of coronary artery spasm in symptomatic and silent myocardial ischaemia. JACC 9: 249—262
45. Maseri A, Chierchia S, Davies G (1986) Pathophysiology of coronary occlusion in acute infarction. Circulation 73: 233—239
46. Maseri A, Severi S, Nes MD et al (1978) Variant angina; one aspect of a continuous spectrum of vasospastic myocardial ischaemia: pathogenetic mechanisms, estimated incidence, clinical and coronary arteriographic findings in 138 patients. Am J Cardiol 42: 1019—1935
47. Nabel EG, Ganz P, Gordon JB, Alexander RW, Selwyn AP (1988) Dilatation of normal and constriction of atherosclerotic coronary arteries caused by the cold pressor test. Circulation 77: 43—52
48. Ridolfi FL, Hutchins GM (1977) The relation between coronary artery lesions and myocardial infarcts; ulceration of atherosclerotic plaques precipitating coronary thrombosis. Am Heart J 93: 468—486
49. Roberts WC, Curry RC, Isner JM et al (1982) Sudden death in Prinzmetal's angina with coronary spasm documented by arteriography: analysis of three necropsy cases. Am J Cardiol 50: 203—210
50. Ross R (1986) The pathogenesis of atherosclerosis — an update. New Engl J Med 314: 488—500
51. Saner HE, Gobel FL, Salomonowitz E. Erlien DA, Edward JE (1985) The disease-free wall in coronary atherosclerosis: Its relation to degree of obstruction. J Am Coll Cardiol 6: 1096—1099
52. Sherman CT, Litvack F, Grundfest W et al (1986) Coronary angioscopy in patients with unstable angina pectoris. New Engl J Med 315: 913—919
53. Shimokawa H, Aarhus LL, Van Houtte PM (1987) Porcine coronary arteries with regenerated endothelium have a reduced endothelial-dependent response to aggregating platelets and serotonin. Cir Res 61: 256—270
54. Singh RN (1984) Progression of coronary atherosclerosis: clues to pathogenesis from serial coronary arteriography. Br Heart J 52: 451—61
55. Stadius ML, Maynard C, Fritz JK et al (1985) Coronary anatomy and left ventricular function in the first twelve hours of acute myocardial infarction: the Western Washington randomized intracoronary streptokinase trial. Circulation 72: 292—301
56. Van Dantiz JM, Becker AE (1986) Sudden cardiac death and acute pathology of coronary arteries. Europ Heart J 7: 987—991
57. Vanhoutte PM, Houston DS (1985) Platelets, endothelium and vasospasm. Circulation 72: 728—734
58. Waller BF (1985) Coronary luminal shape and the arc of disease free wall; morphological observation and clinical relevance. JACC 6: 1100—1101
59. Willerson JT, Campbell WB, Winniford MD et al (1984) Conversion from chronic to acute coronary artery disease speculation regarding mechanisms. Am J Cardiol 54: 1349—1354
60. Wilson RF, Holida MD, White CW (1986) Quantitative angiographic morphology of coronary stenoses leading to myocardial infarction or unstable angina. Circulation 73: 286—293

Authors's address:
Prof. Dr. M. J. Davies
British Heart Foundation
Cardiovascular Pathology Unit
St. George's Hospital School
Cranmer Terrace
London SW 17 ORE, UK

Discussion

DAVIES:

I think this is a very interesting observation and would very much fit in with some of our own observations, for example, if you look into interleukine-2 production by fatty plaques. Interleukine-2 receptors are markedly increased in lipid plaques as compared to fibrous plaques. You and I are on the same line, beginning to see the lipid-rich plaque as being an inflammatory process. It comes back to the fact that in atheromatous plaques we may be seeing two quite different processes, smooth muscle proliferation on one hand, lipids and inflammation on the other hand.

VON ARNIM:

How does age come into play? Are the different types of progression connected with age in some respect? Is it true that younger patients tend to have more lipid-rich plaques and older patients would have more of the, perhaps less dangerous, collagenous plaques?

DAVIES

We never have managed to find any correlation that really tells what is controlling the type of plaque present. All you can say is that if you as a clinician would take a hundred patients with stable angina, and in these hundred patients you will have a small number of whose plaques are very lipid-rich and the majority of the patients will have a mixture of both plaque types. I wish I could tell you what determines the plaque types but I cannot. Age is only a real nuisance to pathologists. You do not study older arteries because they calcify.

MASERI:

One thing has been bothering me for some time and I understand that perhaps you are not in the best position to answer directly from his work, because you fill up the coronaries at a physiological perfusion pressure and then cut them later in sections. So you are perhaps not able from your studies to tell us what is the percentage of the surface of the intima which is covered by so-called raised plaque. Is raised plaque so common and so prevalent in a normal population as some studies seem to indicate or is your opinion different?

DAVIES:

I cannot answer the question because you cannot do it both ways, this is the trouble. It is an interesting question you are asking but I cannot answer it.

GOHLKE:

You told us that the altered fissured plaque has a higher content of macrophages and you implied that they have a closer relation to the fissuring. Could it be that they are a secondary phenomenon after the plaque has fissured?

DAVIES:

Yes, it clearly was suggested that their response to the fissuring is hypothesis. The way we are attacking this hypothesis now, it is possible to take the macrophages out of human plaques. You can collagenase the plaque, you can spin the macrophages out. What I think is going to be the interesting work of the next year or two, is looking at those macrophages taken out of a plaque and seeing what their activity is. If they are all just inert sitting there and doing nothing, then I think you are right, they are probably just a secondary phenomenon. On the other hand if you study these macrophages and find they are highly active in the production of collagenase, that would be a piece of information that would suggest they are actually responsible for removing the collagenous tissue. There is no doubt, an awful lot of plaques that fissure, the amount of collagen present in the cap is low and it is the question whether it was low to start with or whether it is being removed.

APPELS:

You mentioned inflammation of the adventitial nerves, could you expand on that? Is this an inflammation or an activation, or even hyperactivation? And is this a constant state or a passing state?

DAVIES:

Well, let me once declare that I am not a believer in the phenomenon. I merely put it down, because in the literature that concept exists. One trouble with perivascular inflammation in atheroma is that if you look at a vessel, the inflammation is behind the plaque. So the inflammation of the adventitia where the nerves run is actually nowhere near the media that is going to be responsible for tonus variation. In other words, the inflammation is in the wrong place. The other thing is that if you look at the cell in that adventitial inflammatory response, there are very many B- and T-cell lymphocytes. The current belief among many is, that adventitial inflammation is a B-cell response to lipid antigens. The question was asked about secondary phenomena. Most people, I think, would believe that inflammatory infiltrates in the adventitia are, purely a secondary phenomenon. But inflammation around the adventitia could interfere with the nerves.

PATRONO:

Before everyone goes away with the impression that your leucotrien B4 is an established mediator of a progression of thrombosis on plaques and starts measuring a B4 everywhere, would you like to comment about the difference between establishing biosynthetic capacity ex vivo in a tissue and actual production in vivo in terms of eicosanoids and what we would need to do in order to address the issue in vivo.

DE CATERINA:

The answer to this question is that in doing what we did. We actually measured the capability of the vascular tissue to produce B4 under a sort of non-physiological stimulus, or under conditions of mechanical stimulation which may be more relevant to physiologic situation. However, I am completely aware of the limitation of the approach of the capability vs actual production and, therefore, a possible approach to this would be the measurement of the in vivo metabolites of the leucotrienes and this is something which is impossible at the moment and hopefully will be possible in some years with the development of more knowledge about in vivo metabolites of these substances.

KARSCH:

From the clinical point of view and personally performing PTCA's, I would rather prefer to take the hands off patients with lipid-rich plaques. Can you give us an idea how high the percentage of patients is in whom you would expect those really difficult plaques in a mixed population? What would you think, 5% or 10%?

DAVIES:

I do not think I can give any guess as to it at all. I think what may comfort the cardiologist doing angioplasty is the fact that most of the lesions causing very high-grade stenoses will be fibrous. That I think is very lucky. The other thing is that I do not think, necessarily, that a lipid-rich plaque may be quite easy to angioplasty. I think I would have to ask somebody who does angioplasty. To me, if you look at the mechanism of angioplasty, just as long as you get your balloon right across the lesion, you probably shunt the lipid up into the adventitia. And certainly, I have seen post-mortem cases where it looks as if that is precisely that happened, that the contents of the plaque went outwards. I guess the danger of a lipid-rich plaque is if the contents of the plaque go downstream, but I think we have to ask a clinician. There is no way you can tell what the lesion is before you go at it.

KRUCOFF:

I think I would much rather squash a softer plaque than a harder one. I think there is no question as you begin to crank up more and more pressure and see that waist persist on a balloon that one that does finally rupture, those are far more frequently the patients where we have a mechanical flap and a potential complication relative to the patients in whom the waist resolves at a lower pressure.

153

DAVIES:

I think the trouble is, we understand very little about what triggers smooth muscle proliferation. I mean, it may well be that if you go squeezing an atheromatous plaque and rupturing it and spraying lipid all over everything everwhere, that that's a beautiful stimulus for smooth-muscle proliferation.

VON ARNIM:

How sure can we be that the healing of a fissure would always go together with the progression of the stenosis. Could not a lipid-rich plaque just empty and the cap heal down to where it belongs?

DAVIES:

Yes, and I think many patients do that, and there are many patients who get away with these episodes, who obliterate the plaque and are not left with a high-grade stenosis. Histologically, that is quite easy to recognize. You can recognize the original collagenous outline of the plaque, and then the center, where there should be lipid, is filled with young connective tissue. So yes, that is not infrequent, and the patients who are lucky are the ones who do precisely that, and I think that probably they are in the majority.

PATRONO:

Michael, one less appreciated conclusion deriving from your studies is that because plaque fissuring is so comon, and platelets obviously serve an important function in repairing most of these ruptures, and because of the increasing use of antiplatelet agents not only in patients at high risk but also in perfectly healthy individuals, the question would be, what would this anti-platelet therapy once it is diffused in the general population do to the process of physiologic repair of plaque fissuring? And I was wondering whether it would not be possible in your future studies to try and reconstruct the therapeutic usage of aspirin or other anti-platelet agents in the patients that you then see and see whether previous aspirin use makes any difference in the characteristics of the plaques that you see.

DAVIES:

I do not have a lot of experience with animal models, but surely an animal model would tell you that. And there are excellent animal models of deep intimal injury.

PATRONO:

Although not many of those that I know of are really relevant to what aspirin does in humans, because all the animal studies have predicted a completely different use of aspirin than what has been proven to be effective in man. For example, they have predicated the need for using very high doses of aspirin combined with dipyridamol, and that has been shown not to be the case in humans.

DAVIES:

But of course you also raised the question of whether the platelet is the main driver of smooth muscle proliferation, and I think the Swedish group, would begin to say that there are many other factors — endothelial, T-lymphocytes or macrophages — that drive smooth muscle.

154

Leukotriene production by human vascular tissues: possible link between the nature of the atherosclerotic lesions and their clinical activity

R. De Caterina, A. Mazzone, D. Giannessi, R. Sicari, W. Pelosi, G. Lazzerini, A. Azzarà*, R. Forder**, F. Carey**, D. Caruso***, G. Galli***, F. Mosca****

C.N.R. Institute of Clinical Physiology, Pisa, *Medical Clinic I, University of Pisa, **I.C.I. Pharmaceuticals, Macclesfield, UK, ***Institute of Pharmacological Sciences, University of Milan, and ****Institute of Surgical Pathology I, University of Pisa, Italy

Introduction

The idea that angiographic assessment of coronary atherosclerosis is a poor predictor of the occurrence of clinical complications is being appreciated more and more. Over a certain age, atherosclerotic lesions in the coronary arteries become common in humans [1]. Clinical manifestations of coronary artery disease are, on the contrary, relatively uncommon phenomena, sometimes occurring erratically and unpredictably in the patient's life. This is especially true of the most catastrophic clinical complications of coronary artery disease, namely unstable angina, myocardial infarction, and sudden cardiac death. On the other hand, a long established and more understandable relationship exists between the angiographic degree of coronary artery lesions and chronic stable angina. Here, the progressive reduction of coronary reserve as a function of the degree of lumen obstruction can easily explain the occurrence of myocardial ischemia in conditions of an increased myocardial oxygen demand. However, stable angina is rarely an unmanageable situation, and we are mostly faced with the problem of unstable events only loosely correlated with quantitative assessment of lumen reductions. Given the strong evidence still relating the proven mechanisms of "coronary instability" — thrombosis and alterations in the vasomotor tone — to atherosclerotic plaques in the coronary arteries [2—6], one is left with the recognition of the limitations of quantitative assessment of lumen reduction as given by angiography, and with the need to explore qualitative features of the atherosclerotic plaque in search for hints that predict the "activation" of the disease.

The atherosclerotic plaque contains mixtures of cells normally resident within the vessel wall (endothelial cells, smooth muscle cells, fibroblasts), and cells normally not present. These include the atherocytes, possibly derived both from smooth muscle cells and macrophages [7], clearly identifiable macrophages, newly immigrated monocytes, and, occasionally, lymphocytes and neutrophils [7, 8]. Occasionally, mast cell infiltrates, mainly in the adventitia, have been described [9] and correlated with the occurrence of coronary artery spasm.

Most, if not all, of these cell types are biosynthetically active in producing leukotrienes, oxygenated derivatives of arachidonic acid endowed with powerful biological activities [10]. One of these compounds, leukotriene (LT) B4, can increase vascular (endothelial) permeability, and is the most potent chemoattractant known so far [10]. The sulfido-peptide leukotrienes (LTC4, LTD4, LTE4) are potent vasoconstrictors [10]. Therefore the production of these substances might be regarded as a mechanism for plaque progression, via the recruitment of further elements of the white series form the flowing blood, and for the pathogenesis of its clinical manifestations, by increasing vascular tone at critical sites.

In order to verify this hypothesis, the following steps should be undertaken:
1) Demonstrate the presence of the critical enzyme, 5-lipooxygenase, catalyzing the conversion of arachidonic acid into leukotriene precursors, or of leukotrienes themselves, in the vessel wall of atherosclerotic vs normal vessels;
2) Clarify the possible source of leukotrienes and correlate the potential of their production with critically occurring cell types in the atherosclerotic lesions;
3) Demonstrate the ability of this production (at least as far as LTB4 is concerned) to reach the luminal surface of the vessel where biological activity may be exerted on the flowing blood;
4) Demonstrate and quantitate this production in vivo.
This work reports the assessment of the first three of such issues.

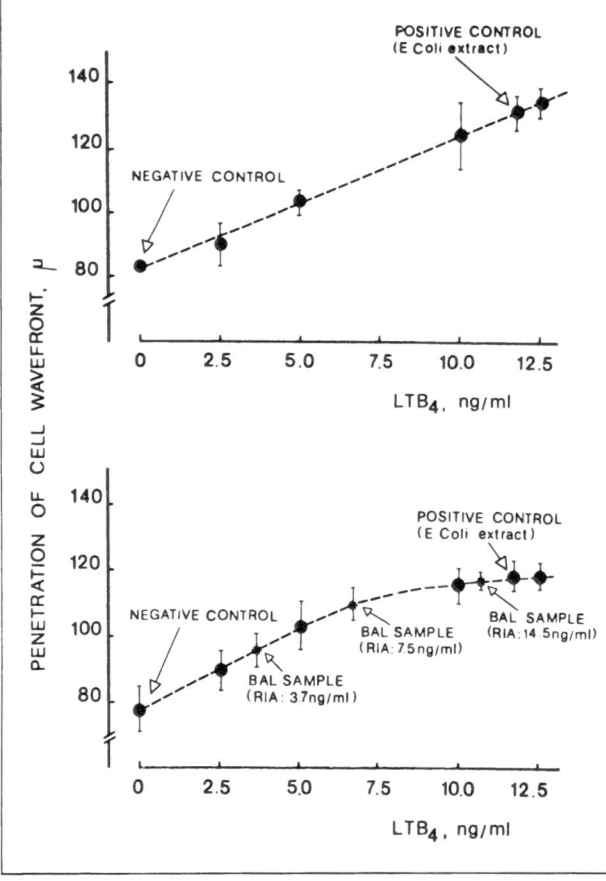

Fig. 1. Upper panel: standard curve of LTB4 bioassay in Boyden chamber. The penetration of the neutrophil wavefront within the Millipore filter of the chamber is shown on the ordinate as a function of LTB4 standard concentration (on the abscissa). The effects of a negative control (buffer) and of a positive control (*Escherichia coli* extract) are also shown. Lower panel: by interpolations of such standard curves, putative LTB4 concentration are attributed to unknown biological samples, in this example derived from broncho-alveolar lavage (BAL) fluid. The unknown samples are also submitted to radioimmunoassay (RIA), with the results indicated. Note the good correlation of the bioassay and RIA results in the unknown samples.

Materials and methods

Human vascular fragments from various sources were obtained during operations of vascular, cardiac, or abdominal surgery. They consisted of aortic fragments, the main source of which were anaeurismectomies, saphenous veins, atrial appendages, and mesenteric arteries. Soon after surgical excision, fragments were placed in tissue culture medium containing newborn calf serum and papaverin; all fragments were processed within three h. Processing consisted of cutting fragments into smaller pieces (average weight, mean $\pm$ SD, 348 $\pm$ 157 mg) and incubating them sequentially at 37 °C, in a Dubnoff shaking water bath: 1) in buffer (Dulbecco's modified phosphate-buffered saline containing calcium and magnesium); 2) in buffer plus ionophore A23187 (IONO) 10—50 µM; 3) in buffer plus arachidonic acid (AA) 25 µM. Incubation times between 5 and 60 min were evaluated. After each step medium was sampled and stored frozen for subsequent eicosanoid determinations. Variants of this protocol included boiling of the fragment to destroy vascular enzymatic activities, or incubations with 5-lipooxygenase inhibitors (nafazatrom 0.5— 5 µg/ml, nordihydro-guaiaretic acid [NDGA] 5—50 µg/ml). Incubations were also performed in chambers (kindly provided by Eric F. Grabowski and Babette B. Weksler, Cornell University Medical College, New York, NY, USA), allowing selective endothelial/adventitial exposure of the fragment to medium. At the end of incubations, fragments were fixed in formalin and destined to histology for plaque classification and semiquantitative assessment of cellularity. Media collected after each incubation step were assayed by specific radioimmunoassays (RIA) for LTB4 and prostacyclin (6-keto-PGF1alpha). LTB4 RIA was validated with two independent techniques: reverse-phase high-performance liquid chromatography (HPLC) and bioassay in Boyden chambers. An excellent agreement was found among the three techniques. An example of this is shown in Fig. 1. However, RIA was the only practicable method for concentrations < 1 ng/ml. RIA sensitivity was (mean $\pm$ SD) 43 $\pm$ 9 pg/ml in the usual assay conditions.

Results

Baseline LTB4 production differed significantly among different tissues (P < 0.01 by analysis of variance), with maximum production observed for fatty and complicated atherosclerotic plaques (Fig. 2).

Production was virtually abolished (> 90% reduction) by boiling of the fragment. Production was increased in the presence of AA and IONO (Fig. 3). Peak of IONO or AA-stimulated production was reached at 20 min in kinetic studies. Both baseline and stimulated productions were decreased dose-dependently in the presence of 5-lipoxygenase inhibitors: for IONO-stimulated production inhibition was (mean $\pm$ SEM) by 60 $\pm$ 7% with nafazatrom 0.5 µg/ml; by 71 $\pm$ 6% with nafazatrom 5 µg/ ml; by 42 $\pm$ 8% with NDGA 5 µg/ml; by 61 $\pm$ 7% with NDGA 50 µg/ml (all P < 0.01). LTB4 production was able to reach the luminal side of the vascular fragments in chamber studies (baseline production for fatty plaques (mean $\pm$ SD, pg/ cm^2 area): 420 $\pm$ 160; with AA: 1035 $\pm$ 950). There was no correlation with concomitantly measured prostacyclin production. Actually, the vascular fragments

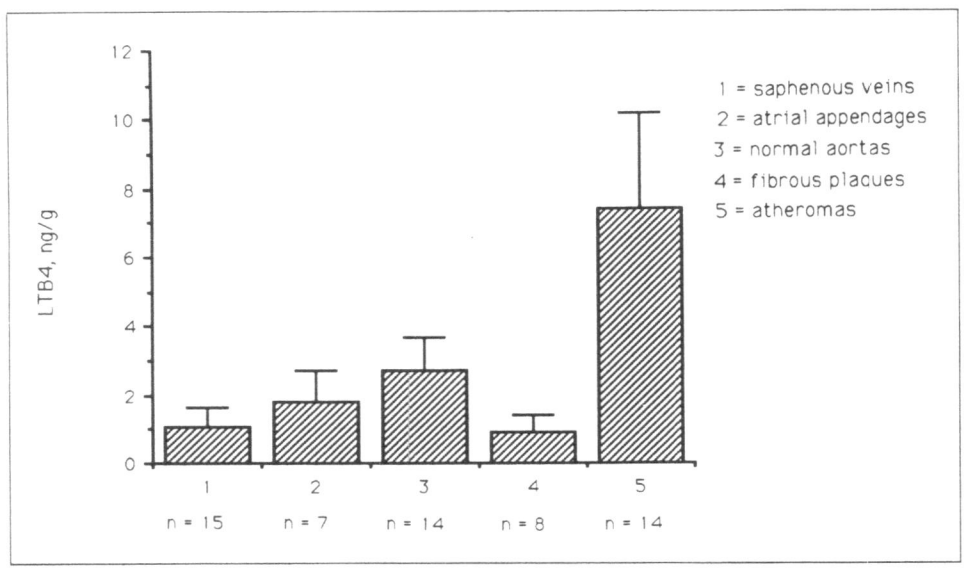

Fig. 2. Basal (unstimulated) LTB4 production (mean ± SD) by different vascular fragments. The greatest production is observed for fatty plaques, the lowest for fibrous plaques.

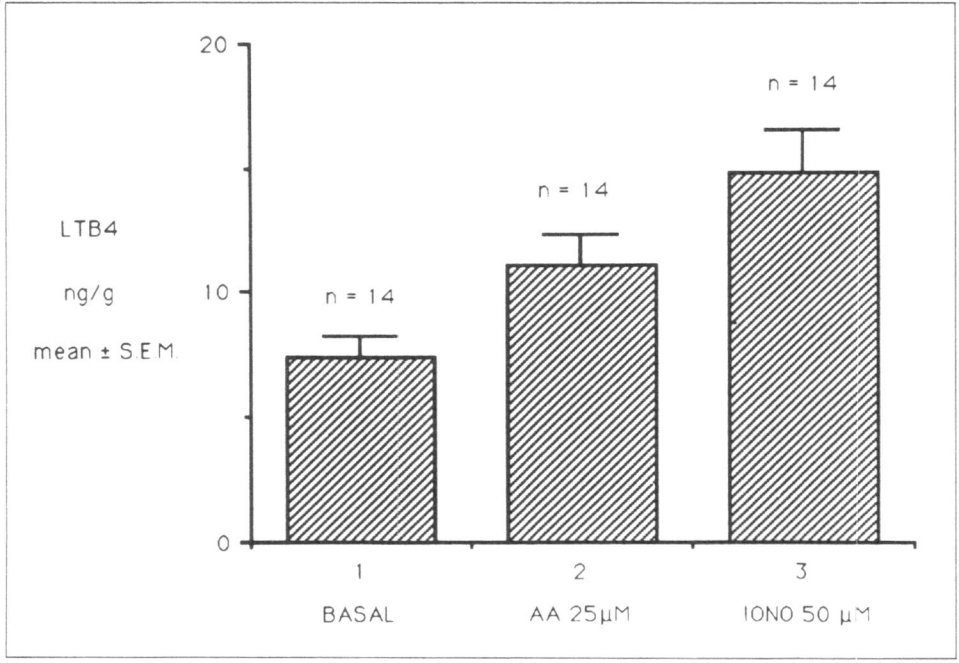

Fig. 3. LTB4 production (mean ± SEM) by human fatty atherosclerotic plaques in basal conditions (mechanical stimulation only) and stimulated conditions (by arachidonic acid (AA)) and calcium ionophore A 23187 (IONO).

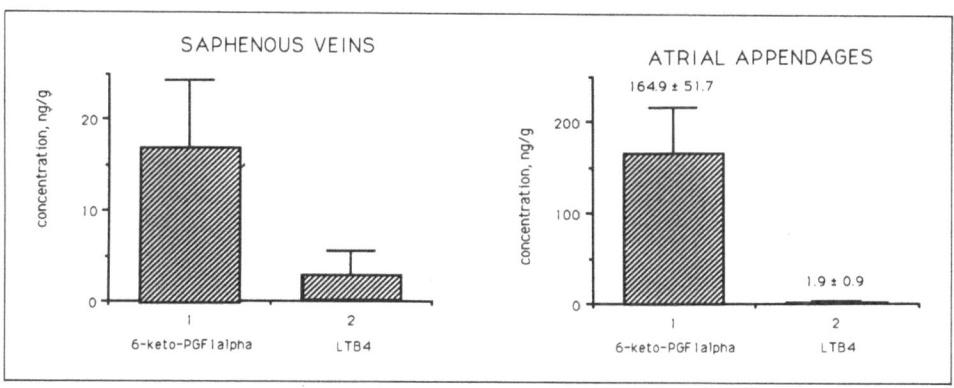

Fig. 4. Compared basal (unstimulated) prostacyclin and LTB4 productions (mean ± SD) by saphenous veins and atrial appendages. These two tissues differ widely in terms of both endothelial surface-to-volume ratio and of prostacyclin production, yet they differ very little for LTB4 production, indicating a putative non-endothelial origin of this last compound.

most active in prostacyclin production, atrial appendages, for which endothelial surface/volume ratio is highest, produced nearly as much as LTB4 as saphenous veins, for which prostacyclin production was much less (Fig. 4). On the contrary, a good correlation (r = 0.85, P < 0.05) was found with the histologic assessment of plaque cellularity for atherosclerotic lesions. Plaque cellularity was also greater in fatty and complicated lesions than in fibrous plaques.

Conclusion

This work demonstrates the existence of a potential for leukotriene production in human vascular tissues. Evidence for the chemical identity of LTB4 with the compound measured by our RIA, besides the antibody specificity, lies, 1) on the stimulability of the production by arachidonic acid, supplying substrate for 5-lipooxygenase, and the ionophore A23187, activating membrane phospholipase(s) subsequent to increase in cytosolic calcium; and 2) on its specific inhibition by compounds such as nafazatrom and NDGA used in a concentration range similar to that reported by others to inhibit 5-lipoxygenase. This is the first such demonstration in human tissues. Previous investigators [11, 12] have shown analogous results in vascular tissues from other species. However, much more relevant to pathophysiologic considerations than a generic vascular potential for leukotriene generation is the demonstration that production is greater in some specific types of atherosclerotic lesions, such as fatty and complicated plaques, and that it correlates with plaque cellularity. This correlation, together with the poor relationship with the presence of endothelium in the fragment — maximum for atria where the high surface-to-volume ratio correlates with the production of a typical endothelial product, prostacyclin [13] — points strongly to a production by the cellular infiltrate of the plaque and not by endothelial cells. Morphologic features of such infiltrates are largely superimposable to what is known to be the usual natural source of leukotrienes in the body [10]. The production of LTB4 in some atherosclerotic lesions due to the potent biologic activity of the compound, can be hypothesized to be related to an accelerated plaque evolution. Leukotriene B4 adds, in this regard, to interleukin 1 [14], platelet-derived growth factor [15], and fibroblast growth factor [16] as a possible mediator of the progression of the plaque, and might mark the presence of white cell infiltrates within the atherosclerotic lesions.

References

1. Baroldi G, Scomazzoni G (1967) Coronary circulation in the normal and the pathologic heart. Office of the Surgeon General, Dept. of the Army. Washington, D.C.
2. Davies MJ, Thomas AC (1985) Plaque fissuring — the cause of acute myocardial infarction, sudden ischemic death and crescendo angina. Br Heart J 53: 363—373
3. De Wood MA, Spores J, Notske R, Mouser LT, Burroughs R, Golden MS, Lang HT (1980) Prevalence of total coronary occlusion during the early hours of transmural myocardial infarction. New Engl J Med 303: 897—902
4. Falck E (1985) Unstable angina with fatal outcome: dynamic coronary thrombosis leading to infarction and/or sudden death. Circulation 71: 699—708
5. Maseri A (1987) Role of coronary artery spasm in symptomatic and silent myocardial ischemia. J Am Coll Cardiol 9: 249—262
6. Maseri A, Chierchia S, Davies G (1986) Pathophysiology of coronary occlusion in acute infarction. Circulation 73: 233—239
7. Ross R (1986) The pathogenesis of atherosclerosis — An update. N Engl J Med 314: 488—500
8. Baroldi G, Giuliano G (1986) Ischemic heart disease: clinical and pathological mismatch. Can J Cardiol July Suppl. A: 248—254
9. Forman MB, Oates JA, Robertson D, Robertson RM, Roberts LJ, Virmani R (1985) Increased adventitial mast cells in a patient with coronary spasm. N Engl J Med 313: 1138—1141
10. Lewis RA, Austen F (1984) The biologically active leukotrienes. Biosynthesis, metabolism, receptors, functions and pharmacology. J Clin Invest 73: 889—897
11. Piper PJ, Letts LG, Galton SA (1983) Generation of a leukotriene-like substance from porcine vascular and other tissues. Prostaglandins 25: 591—599
12. Woelbling RH, Aeringhaus U, Peskar BM, Peskar JA (1983) Release of slow-reacting substance of anaphylaxis from layers of guinea pig aorta. Prostaglandins 25: 823—828
13. De Caterina R, Dorso CR, Tack-Goldman K, Weksler BB (1985) Nitrates and endothelial prostacyclin production: studies in vitro. Circulation 71: 176—182
14. Bevilacqua MP, Pober JS, Wheeler ME, Cotran RS, Gimbrone MA Jr (1985) Interleukin 1 activation of vascular endothelium. Effects on procoagulant activity and leukocyte adhesion. Am J Pathol 121: 394—403
15. Shimokado K, Raines EW, Madtes DK, Barrett TB, Benditt EP, Ross R (1985) A significant part of macrophage-derived growth factor consists of at least two forms of PDGF. Cell 43: 277—286
16. Baird A, Mormede P, Bohlen P (1985) Immunoreactive fibroblast growth factor in cells of peritoneal exudate suggests its identity with macrophage-derived growth factor. Biochem Biophys Res Commun 126: 358—364

Author's address:
Raffaele De Caterina, M. D.
C.N.R. Institute of Clinical Physiology
Via Savi, 8
56100 Pisa, Italy

Preventive strategies for postinfarction patients

P. Mathes

Klinik Höhenried für Herz- und Kreislaufkrankheiten, Bernried, FRG

In coronary heart disease, whether after myocardial infarction, in patients with angina pectoris, or in those with silent myocardial ischemia, the major threat for the patient is the progression of the disease. We must consider that there are two underlying mechanisms that lead to such progression. On the one hand there are rapid phenomena, like platelet aggregation, thrombosis, spasm and changes in vasomotor tone, which may lead to a rapid occlusion within preexisting atherosclerotic lesions. For the development of myocardial infarction and unstable angina, as we have seen, the hallmark is the rupture of the plaque with subsequent thrombus formation. In atherosclerosis the formation of new lesions is slow and independent from the forementioned rapid phenomena. Thus, in secondary prevention, one has to deal with both mechanisms; we must address the rapid phenomena as well as prevent the formation of new lesions, while trying to slow the process of atherosclerosis in general.

Some of the treatment criteria are generally accepted. For example, following myocardial infarction, and other forms of coronary disease, it is necessary for the patients to quit smoking, a recommendation most physicians concur with. The careful observations by Hickey et al. [3] demonstrated that the patient who continues to smoke following his first myocardial infarction will double his risk of dying from the manifestations of the disease in comparison to the one who stops smoking. There seems little reason to debate these observations.

The debate continues about the ideal levels of blood lipids which should be maintained for the patient following myocardial infarction. Recent information indicates that we may have to reconsider the levels of blood lipids recommended for our coronary patients. In an angiographically controlled study Blankenhorn et al. could demonstrate that a substantial reduction of total cholesterol, achieved by the combination of niacin and cholestyramine, also has a substantial impact on the progression of coronary artery disease. In a double-blind, prospective, controlled study, he was able to demonstrate, that a decline in total cholesterol of 25% was able to decrease the occurrence of new lesions by more than 50%. By closely observing the progression of lesions in bypass grafts it was observed that the rate of new closures was not deeply affected. In patients on treatment the occurrence of new lesions could be substantially decreased and the rate of new closures also could be affected in bypass grafts. Thus, the recommended levels in total cholesterol probably have to be set at a much lower point than previously considered.

In an attempt to achieve the optimum in terms of secondary prevention following the first manifestation of coronary artery disease, many physicians and clinics employ a formal exercise program as a means of achieving the desired goal. Previous observations have shown that aside from the influence of medication, exercise will lead to a decrease in the levels of blood lipids, particularly in LDL-cholesterol and may increase the level of HDL-cholesterol, depending on the amount of exercise done per week. An additional factor affecting secondary prevention, the level of the arterial pressure, will not be affected if the pressure is normal to begin with; however, in hypertensive patients, a formal exercise program will lead to a decrease in blood pressure.

In patients with angina pectoris exercise is generally regarded as a therapeutic measure that has beneficial effects aside from the influence on risk factors in regard to secondary prevention. Heart rate and systolic blood pressure will be lower for any given workload, thus enabling the patient to achieve a higher exercise capacity without affecting the myocardial O_2-consumption. Whether or not an endurance training program can affect the angina threshold is still a matter of debate. In a carefully controlled study, Froelicher et al. [2] demonstrated that regular endurance training performed for one year is able to decrease the index of myocardial ischemia as documented by quantitative analysis of a thallium scintigram on exercise, in comparison to those patients who do not regularly exercise for the same period of time. If one considers the progressive nature of the disease and the resulting increase in the ischemia index which will occur in the course of time, the exercise effect is even more remarkable.

In silent myocardial ischemia the recommendation for exercise therapy has been regarded with great skepticism, since patients may exceed their ischemia threshold without noticing any warning signs. In our rehabilitation program we therefore recommend restriction of the exercise intensity to levels well below the submaximal heart reate obtained during the exercise test, in order to avoid the danger of ischemia during endurance training. The recommended heart rate is the resting heart rate plus 60% of the difference between the resting and maximal heart rate, similar to the formula proposed by Karvonen. In order to obtain information about the effects achieved, we examined or patients by quantitative ST-segment analysis during bicycle ergometry before and following an exercise program, of three weeks. The desired heart rate was achieved during a period of endurance training of 20 min per day, five times a week. In the exercise ECG the typical response was observed; at identical workload, the extent of ST-segment-depression was less than prior to the beginning of the endurance training. A typical example shows that with identical exercise intensity, the double product decreased from 31.000 to 26.000, a reduction of 16% in this particular patient. At the same time the ST-depression at the identical load decreased from 3.3 mm to 1.9 mm. Alternatively, for example, at a 4 mm ST-segment-depression, the double product was identical at the begining as well as at the end of the training period. The total load achieved (in other words, the watts multiplied by the minutes), showed a substantial increase, in this case from 625 to 900 watts per min. As an average for our patients, the double product at the peak load decreased from 31.000 ± 6.000 to 26.000 ± 5.000, at an average of 1.200 watts × min. As a consequence of this decline in the double-product, with the consecutive decrease in myocardial oxygen demand, the average ST-segment-depression at the identical workload decreased from 2.8 ± 0.8 to 2.2 ± 0.6 mm, demonstrating the reduced amount of myocardial ischemia.

When one summarizes the endurance training induced changes in patients with silent myocardial ischemia, there is an increase in exercise tolerance, and a decrease of ischemia at identical workloads, in all likelihood a secondary effect due to the decrease of the double product reflecting myocardial oxygen consumption at identical load. Thus, by employing exercise as a means of secondary prevention with the general aim of slowing down the rate of progression of atherosclerosis, the exercising patient will more easily achieve the control of his blood pressure, it may be easier for him to stop smoking, and it will have a favorable effect on lipid levels. The patients sense of well-being may improve, weight problems may improve as well as his ability to cope with stress. Thus, we feel that an intense exercise program can be recommended as a part of the general measures aimed at slowing the progression of coronary artery disease.

References

1. Blankenhorn DH, Nessim SA, Johnson RL (1987) Beneficial effects of combined colestipol-niacin therapy on coronary atherosclerosis and coronary venous bypass grafts. Jama 257: 3233
2. Froelicher V, Jensen D, Genter F et al (1984) A randomized trial of exercise training in patients with coronary heart disease. J Am Med Assoc 252: 1291
3. Hickey N, Mulcahy R et al (1983) Cigar and pipe smoking related to four-year survival of coronary patients. Br Heart J 49: 423
4. Hollmann W (1983) Sport und körperliches Training als Mittel der Präventivmedizin in der Kardiologie. In: Hollmann W, ed. Zentrale Themen der Sportmedizin. Berlin, Springer: 4–9
5. Mathes P (1988) Indications and contraindications of training in angina pectoris. Eur Heart J 9 (Suppl A)

Author's address:
Prof. Dr. P. Mathes
Klinik Höhenried für Herz- und Kreislauferkrankungen
D-8139 Bernried, FRG

Discussion

VON ARNIM:
The degree of ST segment depression that you showed, were these sums of ST depression from different leads or was it one lead showing 4 mm?

MATHES:
The average lead; this was one lead for a 4 mm ST segment depression.

MASERI:
We have done observations similar to yours with repeated exercise testing. There is a lot of data in the literature showing that with the Bruce exercise testing, the exercise time gets longer but heart rate, blood pressure further remains constant. We have also measured total body oxygen consumption indicating the work the individual was doing, and that also remained constant, so the conclusion is, as previously suggested by other authors, when exercise is repeated in the same environment on the same tool, machine, bicycle, ergometer or treadmill the patient learns to work more efficiently.

163

They learn to walk the treadmill at the same speed, the same inclination, consuming less oxygen, and up doing less work. The total body does less work and therefore the heart also does less work. So one component of the training effect is learning how to walk — not necessarily training the heart or the circulation in itself.

MATHES:

The basic training effect is certainly one of adaptation to the instrumentation. In our experience walking on the treadmill is for all patients very difficult and cumbersome and that makes them very anxious, so we relied on using the bicycle ergometer, which for the majority of people is more familiar. Obviously the major impact in exercise tolerance in increase. There are data which show that, for example, if you just train one leg, these are data using muscle biopsies, that you get your increase in the mitochondrial activity in the trained leg and not in the parallel one, which has not been subjected to exercise training, so there is some objective evidence that you improve peripheral oxygen utilization by training, although that has not been proven in this case.

Preventive efficacy of revascularization in unstable angina pectoris

K. R. Karsch

Eberhard Karls-University of Tübingen, Div. of Cardiology, FRG

Introduction

Since the primary description of the prognosis in patients with unstable angina in a 10-year prospective follow-up study in 1973, the treatment has evolved considerably [1]. Reviewing the recent studies regarding unstable angina the interest is focussed on two major themes: first, the newer concepts regarding the mechanisms of unstable angina based on recent pathophysiologic investigations and, secondly, the apparent differences in outcome between the different studies using medical and interventional invasive therapeutic regimens.

The major drawback that makes the clinical application of all the available studies difficult is the inhomogenous definition of unstable angina resulting in heterogeneous patient populations. It seems questionable if statification in low and high risk subsets as suggested by Fahri et al. can solve this problem, since the basic definition is not affected [2]. Independent of the response to vigorous medical therapy it is useful for an interventional trial to assure a homogeneous study group and include the requirement of transient ST-T changes in the electrocardiogram [3] although by no means all patient with this syndrome will demonstrate electrographic changes on admission [4, 5, 6].

Secondly, histologic sectioning of the coronary arteries in patients with unstable angina has revealed that rupture, cracking, and ulceration of the majority of sclerotic plaques have associated mural or occlusive thrombi [7, 8, 9, 10].

Thus, current recommendations for the management of unstable angina include hospitalization and intensive treatment with nitrates, beta-blockers, calcium-antagonists, aspirin and/or IV heparin [11, 12].

Although in the majority of patients a satisfactory response can be achieved initially (low risk group) [13], pure medical therapy does not prevent reoccurance with subsequent myocardial infarction and sudden death during the early follow-up [1, 13]. Additionally, attempts to improve prognosis with surgical interventions have been proven unsatisfactory. Although it has been shown in prospective and randomized studies that the incidence of recurrent ischemic syndroms is reduced by early bypass surgery, these studies failed to demonstrate a benefit for surgery in terms of morbidity and mortality [14, 15].

An alternative interventional approach is provided by percutaneous transluminal angioplasty in patients with unstable angina pectoris [16, 17, 18, 19]. The early results of angioplasty in patients with one vessel coronary artery disease indicate an acceptable risk-benefit ratio [17, 18, 19]. The role of angioplasty in patients with multivessel disease has yet not been clarified.

Thus, the purpose of the still ongoing study was to assess the actual mortality and morbidity in a group of unselected patients with unstable angina and multivessel disease in whom vigorous medical therapy failed and angioplasty and/or bypass surgery were used complementary for the further therapeutic management.

Patients and methods

Between April 1985, and June 1987, the data of 113 consecutive patients were analyzed retrospectively. All patients satisfied the following criteria:
1) Chest pain at rest for at least 15 min on admission consistent with myocardial ischemia;
2) Recurrance of angina pectoris despite maximal medical therapy, sedation and bed rest for at least 24 h;
3) Reversible ST segment or T-wave abnormalities;
4) No evidence for definite myocardial necrosis (CPK less than twice normal, no Q wave development);
5) Coronary two- or three-vessel disease on emergency angiography after the first 24 h of medical therapy.

Excluded from the retrospective analysis were patients not suitable for either angioplasty or bypass surgery. All patients were monitored in the coronary care unit. Initial treatment included administration of beta-adrenergic blockers, calcium-antagonists and intravenous nitroglycerin. Additionally, all patients were on intravenous heparin to prolong thrombintime at least twice than normal and 250 mgs of aspirin daily. All patients remained unstable and had emergency angiography within the next 24 h.

In patients designated for percutaneous transluminal angioplasty dilatation was performed immediately after the diagnostic catheterization. Only the ischemia-related vessel was dilated. The ischemia-related vessel was identified by the correlation of the electrocardiographic changes during the anginal attack with the angiographic finding. Changes in the electrocardiogramm in the precordial leads V_1-V_5 were related to coronary artery lesions of the left anterior descending artery while electrocardiographic changes in II, III and aVF reflected the right coronary artery and changes in I and V_5, V_6 lesions in the circumflex artery. The angiograms were performed in multiple routine angulations and interpreted independently by two experienced cardiologists. A more then 50% reduction of lumen diameter was defined as a significant stenosis. Biplane cineangiograms were analyzed to determine left ventricular volumes and function and analysis of wall motion abnormalities.

Angioplasty was performed after additional premedication of a bolus of 5 000 U of heparin and sublingual nifedipine (10 mgs). A mean of three inflation periods was used with an inflation pressure up to 10 atmospheres. Percutaneous transluminal angioplasty was considered successful if the lumen diameter of the stenosis was reduced to less than 50%. All patients were monitored for at least 24 h by the coronary care unit after the procedure. In all patients a surgical team stood by for emergency bypass grafting.

In patients designated for primary aorto coronary bypass grafting, surgery was performed within the next 24 h. The patients were transferred from the cadiac care unit directly to the operating room.

Endpoint of the study was on hospital admission. A peri- or postinterventional myocardial infarction was diagnosed when new Q-waves developed in the 12-lead electrocardiogram with an increase of CPK and CPKMB more than twice than normal. Decision either for performing percutaneous transluminal coronary angioplasty or bypass surgery was based on the following exclusion cirteria for angioplasty:

1) left ventricular ejection fraction less than 30%;
2) left main stem stenosis equal or more than 50%
3) in three-vessel disease: stenosis of more than 90% in both non-ischemia related coronary arteries.

Although in six patients surgery was rejected because of severe peripheral coronary artery disease, in these patients angioplasty was performed because of otherwise intractable angina at rest. The patients are not included in this retrospective study.

Results

The primary success rate of percutaneous transluminal coronary angioplasty in patients with two- and three-vessel disease was 82% (56 of 68). The success rate in patients with two-vessel disease was 89% (40 of 45 patients) and thus considerable higher than in patients with three-vessel disease with 70% (16 of 23 patients) (Fig. 1). Emergency bypass operation was neccessary in seven patients. Two of these

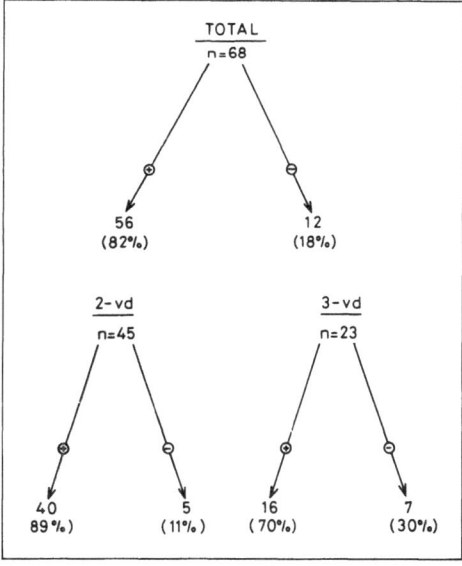

Fig. 1. Success rate of acute PTCA in patients with unstable angina and multivessel disease. The success rate in patients with two-vessel disease is comparable to patients with stable angina. In three-vessel disease, however, the primary success rate is reduced.

patients had two-vessel and five three-vessel disease. Nevertheless, four patients developed a myocardial infarction, one of the patients with two-vessel disease and three with three-vessel disease.

Percutaneous transluminal coronary angioplasty of the left anterior descending artery had a success rate of 70% (30 of 43 vessels). In the eight patients with an ischemia-related circumflex artery the success rate was 88% and in 12 patients, in whom the right coronary artery was the dilated vessel success rate was 83% (10 of 12 vessels). In 12 of the 68 patients percutaneous transluminal coronary angioplasty was unsuccessful. Attempts to cross the subtotal lesion (three patients) or total occlusion (one patient) with the balloon catheter (although the guide wire could pass the lesion in three of these patient) was the cause of failure. One of the four patients developed acute angina and signs of reocclusion after the procedure and was immediately transferred to surgery, the other three were operated within the next 6 to 12 h.

In the remaining eight patients in whom angioplasty was not successful, reocclusion or restenosis with angina and ST-segment or T-wave changes occurred within 30 min up to 2 h after primary successful transluminal coronary angioplasty. Although reangioplasty was initiated immediately percutaneous transluminal angioplasty failed to reopen the vessel persistently in two patients and subsequent emergency surgery was necessary in both patients. In one patient with two-vessel disease and reocclusion, bypass surgery was not performed although myocardial infarction evolved since the ischemia-related vessel was a non-dominant circumflex artery.

From eight patients who demonstrated signs of reocclusion, in six Patients emergency bypass grafting was performed acutely. One patient of the total group of patients treated with transluminal angioplasty died early postoperatively due to an extensive myocardial infarction and cardiologic shock. He had a two-vessel disease with a subtotal proximal lesion of the left anterior descending artery and a 70% stenosis of the right coronary artery. Thus, mortality of patients designated for angioplasty was 1.5% with a morbidity, i.e., occurence of myocardial infarction of 13%.

In 45 patients primary aorto coronary bypass surgery was performed according to the above mentioned criteria with a mean of 3.6 grafts per patient.

Twelve patients had a significantl lesion of the left main stem and the other 37 patients had severe three-vessel disease. In eight patients a transmural myocardial infarction occurred peri- or postoperatively.

Five patients died during the early postoperative period. Thus, mortality in this group was 11% and morbidity 17%. For the total group of 113 patients, in-hospital mortality was 5.3% (six of 113 patients) and occurence of transmural myocardial infarction was 11.5% (13 of 113 patients).

Discussion

The rather strict criteria for unstable angina with the inclusion of electrocardiographic ST-segment of T-wave changes used in this study and the criteria of persistent intermittent chest pain despite maximal vigorous medical therapy stratifies this study group in the high risk subset of patients with unstable angina pectoris [11,

12]. In this subset of patients aggressive management is required because of the increased risk of an ultimate myocardial infarction and sudden death [20, 21, 22]. Since the majority of patients with unstable angina have multivessel disease [18, 19] evaluation of the clinical value of percutaneous transluminal coronary angioplasty is of special interest. In patients with single vessel disease angioplasty compares favorably with aorto coronary bypass surgery in patients with unstable angina [17]. In patients with coronary multivessel disease, however, both methods seems to have their special indications and thus are complementary approaches in the routine clinical setting. In this special subgroup angioplasty seems to be an appropriate method in selected patients to stabilize a patient's condition even though no "complete" revascularization can be achieve in the acute setting. Thus, dilatation of the ischemia-related artery stabilizes most patients and morbidity and mortality of bypass surgery in the acute stage of unstable angina can be avoided [23].

The primary success rate of percutaneous transluminal coronary angioplasty in patients with two-vessel disease is with 89% comparable to patients with one-vessel disease with or without unstable angina [16, 24]. Success rate in patients with three-vessel disease in the acute stage, however, is considerably reduced. This is partially due to the increased technical difficulties in passing the critical stenosis in diffuse diseased vessels with the balloon catheter. In all patients in whom the crossing was impossible even super low profile balloons did not improve success. The ultimate outcome in patients with three-vessel disease treated with angioplasty was a result of extensive sclerotic changes in the proximal segments of the ischemia-related artery and the technical limitations of the dilatation device. Due to these limitations, complication rate in these patients was considerably higher than in patients with two-vessel disease and in comparison to the report of de Feyter et al. [24], and substantially higher than the 3% complication rate reported for elective procedures [25]. This may additionally be related to the severe clinical unstable condition of the high risk subset of our patients.

The complication rate of the 45 patients designed to primary bypass surgery with a mortality of 11% is comparable to the results of other studies [25]. The pooled complication rate of this retrospective clinical study demonstrate the improved preventive efficacy in the management of patients with severe unstable angina by angioplasty.

The morbidity of patients with three-vessel disease demonstrates, however, that the selection of patients designated for treatment with angioplasty is crucial. Even though patients with severe left main stem or three vessel disease and impaired left ventricular function were selected for bypass surgery, angioplasty has a clearly higher risk and a reduced primary success rate. Due to the limited number of patients we could not arrive at specific determinants for selection of patients in this subgroup. Further clinical studies are necessary to identify those patients with three-vessel disease in whom angioplasty may reduce morbidity in the acute phase of the unstable syndrom.

References

1. Gazes PC, Mobley EM jr., Duncan RC, Humphries GB (1973) Preinfarction (unstable) angina — a prospective study — ten year follow up prognostic significance of electrocardiographic changes. Circulation 48: 331—337
2. Farhi JJ, Cohen M, Fuster V (1986) The broad spectrum of unstable angina pectoris and its implications for future controlled trials. Am J Cardiol 58: 547—550
3. Smitherman T (1986) Unstable angina pectoris: The first half century: natural history, pathophysiology and treatment. Am J of Med Sciences 292: 395—406
4. Beamish RE, Storrie VM: Impending myocardial infarction: Recognition and management. Circulation 21: 1107—1115, 1960
5. Krauss, KR, Hutter AM jr., De Sanctis RW (1972) Acute coronary insufficiency: course and follow up. Arch Intern Med 129: 808—813
6. Lopes MG, Spivac AP, Harrison DC, Schröder JS (1974) Prognosis in coronary care unit non-infarction cases. JAMA 228: 1558—1562
7. Falk E (1983) Plaque rupture with severe pre-existing stenosis precipitating coronary thrombosis: Characteristics of coronary atherosclerosic plaques underlying occlusive thrombi. Br Heart J 50: 127—134
8. Falk E (1985) Unstable angina with fatal outcome: dynamic coronary thrombosis leading to infarction and sudden death. Circulation 71: 699—708
9. Davies MJ, Thomas AC (1984) Thrombosis and acute coronary artery lesions in sudden cardiac ischemic death. N Engl J Med 310: 1137—1140
10. Davies MJ, Thomas AC (1985) Plaque fissuring — The cause of acute myocardial infarction, sudden ischemic death, and crescendo angina. Br Heart J 53: 363—373
11. Cohen M, Fuster V (1986) Unstable angina: Is it time for more aggressive therapy? Eur Heart J 7: 1014—1015
12. Hugenholtz PG (1986) Unstable angina revisted once more. Eur Heart J 7: 12
13. Bertolasi CA, Tronge JE, Riccitelli MA, Villamayor RM, Zuffardi E (1976) Natural history of unstable angina with medical or surgical therapy. Chest 70: 596—605
14. Unstable angina pectoris study group (1978) Unstable angina pectoris: national cooperative study group to compare surgical and medical therapy. II. In-hospital experience and initial follow up results in patients with one, two and three vessel disease. Am J Cardiol 42: 839—848
15. Brown CA, Hutter AM, De Sanctis RW (1981) Prospective study of medical and urgent surgical therapy in randomisable patients with unstable angina pectoris: results of in-hospital and chronic mortality and morbidity. Am Heart J 102: 959—964
16. Williams DO, Riley RS, Singh AK, Gerwitz H, Most AS (1981) Evaluation of the role of coronary angioplasty in patients with unstable angina pectoris. Am Heart J 102: 1—9
17. Meyer J, Schmitz HJ, Kisslich T (1983) Role of percutaneous transluminal coronary angioplasty in patients with stabel and unstable angina pectoris: analysis of early and late results. Am Heart J 106: 973—980
18. Faxon DP, Detre KM, McCable CH. et al (1983) Role of percutaneous transluminal coronary angioplasty in the treatment of unstable angina. Report of the National Heart, Lung and Blood Institute percutaneous transluminal coronary angioplasty and coronary artery surgery study registries. Am J Caridol 53: 131—135
19. De Feyter PJ, Serruys PW, van den Brand M. et al (1985) Emergency coronary angioplasty in refractory unstable angina. N Engl J Med 313: 342—346
20. Cairus JA, Fantus IG, Klassen GA (1976) Unstable angina pectoris. Am Heart J 92: 373—386
21. Plotnick GD (1979) Approach to the management of unstable angina. Am Heart J 98: 243—255
22. Silverman KJ, Grossman W (1984) Angina pectoris: Natural history and strategies for evaluation and management. N Engl J Med 30: 1712—1717
23. Smith CW, Hornway CA, Sutton JP, Allen WB, Yarbrough JW, Tarner J (1985) Emergency and elective surgical intervention for failed PTCA after unstable angina. Im Hugenholtz PG, Goldman BS (Ed.): Unstable angina. Current concepts and management (Schattauer: 1985, 265)
24. de Feyter PJ, Suerreuys PW, Arnold A, Sinoous ML, Wigns W, Genskens R, Soward A, van den Brand M, Hugenholtz PG (1986) Coronary angioplasty of the unstable angina related vessel in patients with multivessel disease. Eu Heart J 7: 460—467

25. Bredlau CE, Roubin GS, Leimgruber PP, Douglas JS, King SB, Grüntzig AR (1985) In hospital morbidity and mortality in patients undergoing elective coronary angioplasty. Circulation 72: 1044—1052
26. National Cooperative Study Group to compare surgical and medical therapy. II. in hospital experience and initial follow-up results in patients with one, two and three vessel disease. Am J Cardiol 48: 517—523 (1981)

Authors' address:
Priv.-Doz. Dr. K. R. Karsch, M.D.
Medical Clinic of the
University of Tuebingen
Abteilung III
Otfried-Mueller-Str. 10
7400 Tübingen, FRG

Discussion

ANDRESEN:

Dr. Karsch, if I understood you correctly, there were differences between the success rate of PTCA of the LAD in those patients who had a two-vessel disease in contrast to those who had a three-vessel disease. What do you think is the reason for not being successful only in dilatating one vessel in a patient who had a two-vessel and in a patient with a three-vessel disease?

KARSCH:

In answer to this question, I would refer to the discussion this morning with Dr. Davies; I think if you have a patient with triple-vessel disease, the atherosclerotic process has involved more of the vessel, which we cannot see. That means that you have in these patients near the left main stem a stenosis of 50% and in the LAD, but the ischemia-related stenosis may be in the second part of the vessel with a 90% stenosis. Although the device has been improved during the last years and the balloons have become better, you will have difficulties to reach the stenosis and then to pass it, there are diffuse disease in the whole proximal parts of the vessel will reduce the success rate.

KRUCOFF:

I would certainly applaud Dr. Karsch' definitions in this case of unstable angina in the patient population. I think you truly have collected a population of very high-risk individuals. My one word of caution, especially in regards to the previous question, would be though that with small numbers, as we all know, in angioplasty experience, things tend to come not evenly distributed but wax and wane; we look at endpoint events of 2% or 8% incidence. For instance, we completed a 300-patient experience with no emergency operations and in the subsequent weeks did four emergency operations. The numbers even themselves out, but I think we have to, as Prof. Maseri was saying earlier, stick with the fact and at the same time, delay interpretations, perhaps of why performance in the LAD and in a small group, looks worse with three-vessel than two-vessel. We have to reserve our interpretations to some degree and be cautious in how we take them until large numbers are available. In larger experiences, not with these patients but with chronic multivessel disease patients, success rates in individual anatomic locations have been rather comparable between two- and three-vessel disease and I would at least urge some caution in taking small subgroups out of this whole group you have collected of these very unstable patients and trying to push the interpretation too far.

KARSCH:

I hope I was clear enough in saying that it is a dangerous business and, of course, you cannot randomize such a study because those are complementary methods and I know, of course, we ourselves do enough PTCA in multivessel disease in stable patients, there is, and that was my point, there is quite a difference and the problem is that in those high risk subgroups mortality is extremely high. It is somewhere between 10%—15% in a normal clinical setting and we have to define the patient with triple-vessel disease in whom we can dilate with a low risk. For that, of course, you need a larger group of patients.

Anti-ischemic therapy with nisoldipine

P. Deeg, K. H. Weiss*, and H. Schmitz*

Deegenbergkurklinik für Innere Krankheiten und des Bewegungsapparates,
AHB-Klinik für Herz- und Kreislauferkrankungen, Bad Kissingen, FRG,
* Bayer AG, Leverkusen, FRG

Introduction

Nisoldipine is a new 1,4-dihydropyridine derivative with a potent vasodilatory and anti-ischemic effect [1—6]. Similar to nifedipine nisoldipine it preferentially binds to the inactivated calcium channel and inhibits transmembrane calcium entry [6]. From this results a negative inotropic action which is, however, 100—1000 times lower in nisoldipine than in nifedipine [6]. In in vitro experiments the duration of inhibition of vascular contractions is nearly three times longer for nisoldipine than that of nifedipine [6]. Nisoldipine shows a 100-times higher vascular selectivity than nifedipine [5, 6]. Therefore, nisoldipine seems to be preferentially suited for the treatment of hypertension and CHD, especially that of vasospastic origin [1—4].

Patients and methods

The study was biometrically planned and its design is shown in Fig. 1. Of the 24 patients originally scheduled to be included and the 26 patients finally included in the study, the results of only 12 patients who had completed all the treatment periods could be assessed. The 12 who were assessed with respect of efficacy were on the average of 53.1 ± 7.2 years old, weighed 77.8 ± 8.1 kg, and were 170.8 ± 4.3 cm tall. One patient was female.

The median duration of the disease was 20 months (1 month — 10 years). The median frequency of angina pectoris attacks was 6—7 per week before the start of treatment.

In the case fo the remaining 12 patients the study was stopped prematurely due to the occurrence of subjective side effects (mostly at the start of treatment) which mainly originated in the pharmacodynamic profile of the test substance or could be interpreted as symptoms of the underlying disease.

Exercise studies were carried out for each patient on the bicycle ergometer upon inclusion in the trial (following a treatment-free preliminary phase of the last three days) and then at the end of each three-week, double-blind, randomized treatment period. These studies were always carried out at 11.00 hrs, 3 h after the ingestion of the morning tablet.

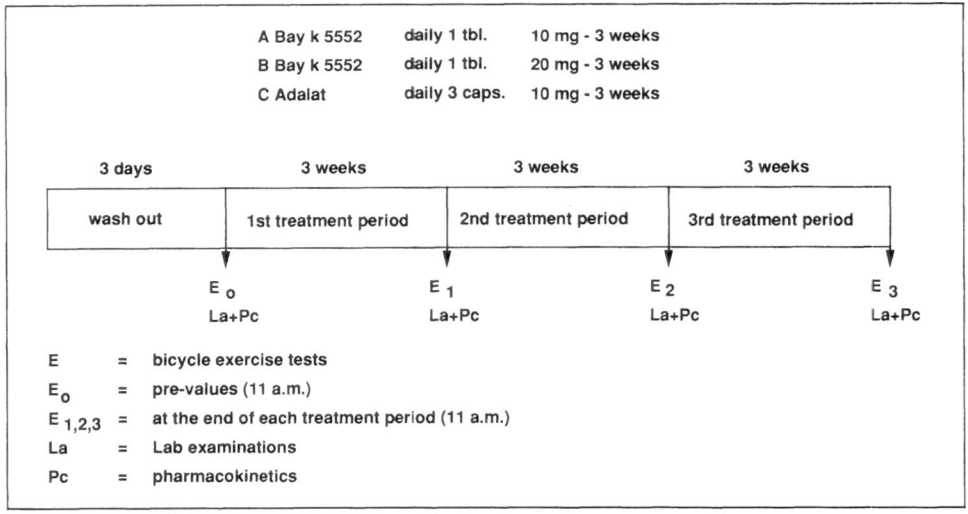

Fig. 1. Study-design: double-blind (double dummy) cross-over study, three treatment periods

Results

All three treatments had a marked anti-ischemic effect, expressed as a reduction in the ST-segment depression at the corresponding maximum exercise level (Table 1; Fig. 2). The exercise tolerance (W × min) showed an increase under all treatment, (Table 2). There was no change in heart rate (Table 3), but there was an obvious decrease in systolic and diastolic blood pressure (Tables 4, 5).

The frequency of angina pectoris attacks (Table 6) decreased noticeably during the three treatment periods, in parallel with the improvement in the ergometric results on the bicycle. Surprisingly, the nitroglycerin tablet consumption did not decrease.

The laboratory tests carried out in order to assess drug tolerance GOT, GPT, alkaline phosphatase, gamma-GT, bilirubin, creatinine, hemoglobin, erythrocytes, leukocytes, and thrombocytes showed, with an exception of two parameters (patients 16 and 26), no deviations from prior values beyond the normal physiological variation. The majority of the 26 patients recorded subjective side effects either once or several times which can mainly be interpreted as an expression of the vasodilating effect of the test substances (Tables 7 and 8).

Conclusion

Similar to other investigators [1, 2] we found a convincing improvement of exercise tolerance, reduction in the frequency of angina pectoris attacks, decrease in elevated

174

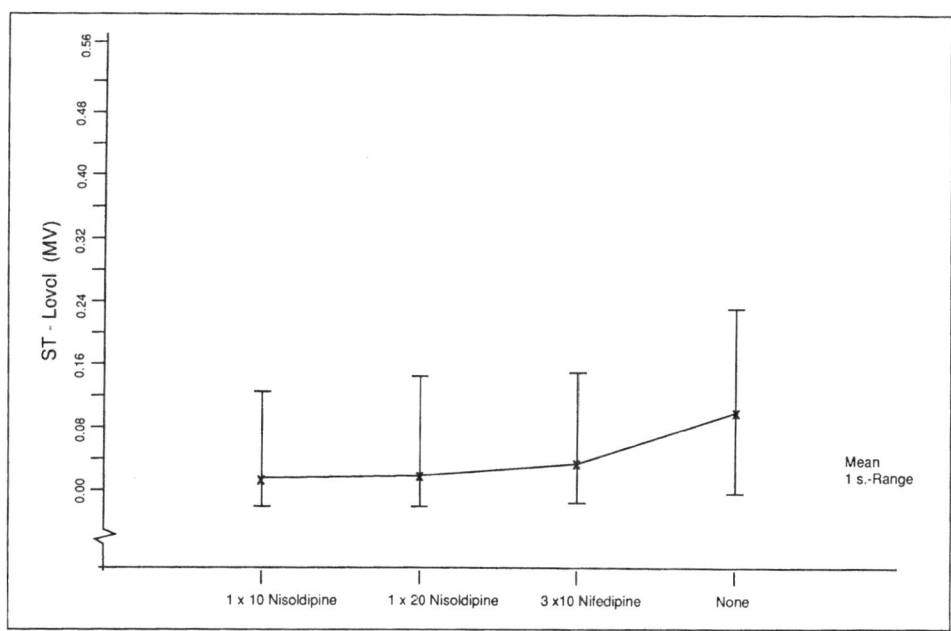

Fig. 2. Reduction of ST-segment depression at maximal load

Table 1: ST-depression [mV], mean ± sd, geometric mean/geometric sd retransformed mean.

exercise step	none	Nisoldipine		Nifedipine 3 × 10 mg
		1 × 10 mg	1 × 20 mg	
max load	0.100 (0.013, 0.242)	0.024 (0.000, 0.122)	0.030 (0.000, 0.139)	0.048 (0.000, 0.142)
1st min recovery	0.096 (0.000, 0.273)	0.030 (0.000, 0.106)	0.030 (0.000, 0.139)	0.056 (0.000, 0.142)
3 rd min recovery	0.065 (0.000, 0.228)	0.016 (0.000, 0.071)	0.033 (0.000, 0.114)	0.040 (0.000, 0.163)
6th min recovery	0.048 (0.000, 0.147)	0.011 (0.000, 0.045)	0.030 (0.000, 0.106)	0.055 (0.000, 0.191)

Table 2: Exercise tolerance [W × min], geometric means geometric sd.

none		Nisoldipine				Nifedipine 3 × 10 mg	
		1 × 10 mg		1 × 20 mg			
555	1.96	618	1.36	653	1.62	647	1.43

175

Table 3: Heart rate [s/min] mean ± sd; geometric mean, geometric sd retransformed mean.

exercise step	none	Nisoldipine		Nifedipine 3 × 10 mg
		1 × 10 mg	1 × 20 mg	
at rest	80 ± 14	76 ± 13	88 ± 14	80 ± 14
max load	126 ± 18	120 ± 13	126 ± 16	128 ± 12
1st min recovery	118 ± 29	119 ± 27	126 ± 25	119 ± 24
3rd min recovery	98 ± 27	96 ± 20	105 ± 20	99 ± 24
6th min recovery	91 ± 17	87 ± 12	97 ± 15	91 ± 12

Table 4: RR systolic [mm Hg] mean ± sd; geometric mean, geometric sd retransformed mean.

exercise step	none	Nisoldipine		Nifedipine 3 × 10 mg
		1 × 10 mg	1 × 20 mg	
at rest	147 ± 19	136 ± 28	131 ± 14	135 ± 12
max load	204 ± 30	188 ± 29	190 ± 35	194 ± 2c
1st min recovery	181 ± 22	166 ± 27	157 ± 28	167 ± 2n
3rd min recovery	165 ± 25	153 ± 27	144 ± 18	156 ± 23
6th min recovery	150 ± 18	134 ± 19	134 ± 20	139 ± 17

Table 5: RR diastolic [mm Hg] mean ± sd; geometric mean, geometric sd retransformed mean.

exercise step	none	Nisoldipine		Nifedipine 3 × 10 mg
		1 × 10 mg	1 × 20 mg	
at rest	95 ± 10	94 ± 13	89 ± 10	93 ± 9
max load	115 ± 16	101 ± 12	102 ± 16	106 ± 12
1st min recovery	101 ± 10	90 ± 11	85 ± 14	93 ± 14
3rd min recovery	93 ± 19	91 ± 7	85 ± 14	91 ± 11
6th min recovery	93 ± 9	92 ± 8	84 ± 15	92 ± 12

Table 6: Angina pectoris attacks/week, nitro consumption/week retransformed means.

	none	Nisoldipine		Nifedipine 3 × 10 mg
		1 × 10 mg	1 × 20 mg	
A.p.-attacks	7.2 (2.00, 15.6)	2.8 (0.02, 12.1)	2.8 (0.00, 10.6)	1.7 (0.01, 7.4)
Nitroglycerin consumption	3.2 (0.05, 11.1)	3.8 (0.16, 18.6)	4.6 (0.17, 22.2)	1.7 (0.02, 7.6)

Table 7: Side effects.

event	prev.	Nisoldipine		Nifedipine 3 × 10 mg
		1 × 10 mg	1 × 20 mg	
A.p.-attacks		4	2	1
pressure left thorax			1	
palpitation	1	3	5	
tachycardia	1	1	2	3
HF increase			1	
heat flutter			1	
dizziness		5	4	2
headache		3	1	1
excited		1		
tinnitus		1		
shortness of breath		1		
outbreak of sweat		1	1	
heartburn	1	1		
edema legs			1	
redness legs			1	
itching			1	
hypotony	1			
exanthema, head		1		
allergy			1	
flush			2	
nausea		1	1	
impaired vision				1
impaired taste		1		
diarrhea				1

Table 8: Side effects.

Treatment	Total	Without	Period	Total	Without
1 × 10 mg Nisoldipine	17	6	pre	26	23
1 × 20 mg Nisoldipine	19	6	1.	24	6
3 × 10 mg Nifedipine	18	11	2.	16	7
			3.	14	10

blood pressure, and ST-segment depression [3, 4]. In contrast to other investigators we saw a surprisingly high rate of side effects [2, 3], which may result from the special conditions under which we carried out our study.

Contrary to the diminution of the frequency of angina pectoris attacks we saw no decrease in nitroglycerin tablet consumption. We believe that patients were able to judge angina pectoris attacks but because of the side effects (Table 7, 8) patients were afraid of having heart attacks and took prophylactic nitroglycerin tablets. But the results of the study underline the marked anti-ischemic and anti-hypertensive effect of nisoldipine. We could show that there were no statistical differences in effect between the lower and higher dosage of nisoldipine or nifedipine treatments. So nisoldipine therapy with a single daily dose of 10 mg seems to be equivalent to nifedipine therapy with three 10 mg-capsules per day. While the anti-ischemic effect is guaranteed, nisoldipine therapy of CHD patients delivers a lower substance load than nifedipine.

References

1. Broustet JP, Pic A (1987) Assessment and comparison of single and double dose of nisoldipine in the prevention of exercise-induced ischaemia — match with sublingual nitroglycerin. In: Hugenzholtz PG, Meyer J (eds) Nisoldipine 1987. Springer, Berlin—Heidelberg—New—York, p 256—262
2. Cagatay M, Frost N, Weiss KH, Wiesner K (1987) Assessment of Long-Term Efficacy and Tolerability of Nisoldipine by the Clinical Data Pool. In: Hugenholtz PG, Meyer J (eds) Nisoldipine 1987. Springer, Berlin—Heidelberg—New York, p 201—209
3. Deeg P, Weiss KH, Schmitz H (1987) Anti-Ischemic Effect of Nisoldipine in Patients with Stable Angina Pectoris. In: Hugenholtz PG, Meyer J (eds) Nisoldipine 1987. Springer Berlin— Heidelberg—New York, p 244—248
4. Deeg P, Weiss KH, Schmitz H (1987) Nisoldipin in der Therapie der essentiellen Hypertonie. Dtsch Med Wschr 112: 433—433
5. Godfraind T, Egleme C, Finet M, Debande B, Jaumin P (1987) Comparison of Nifedipine and Nisoldipine on Human Arteries and Human Cardiac Tissues In Vitro. In: Hugenholtz PG, Meyer J (eds) Nisoldipine 1987. Springer, Berlin—Heidelberg—New York, p 36—44
6. Kazda S, Stasch J-P, Hirth C (1987) Experimental Pharmacology of Nisoldipine: Perspectives from Long-Term Studies. In: Hugenholtz PG, Meyer J (eds) Nisoldipine 1987. Springer Berlin— Heidelberg—NewYork, p 3—12

Authors' address:
Prof. Dr. med. P. Deeg
Deegenbergkurklinik
f. Innere Krankheiten
Burgstraße 21
8780 Bad Kissingen, FRG

Discussion

LEMMER:

The number of side effects is rather high, so could you further comment which kind of side effects were predominant in your 12 patients?

DEEG:

Predominant were headache and dizziness and flush. It was mostly told by the patients.

FOX:

Of the 24 patients, how many of them developed increasingly severe angina or acute myocardial infarction?

DEEG:

There was no myocardial infarction, no heavy side effects, and no deterioration of the clinical situation.

LEMMER:

You mention that nifedipine was equally effective and the number of side effects in your study of nisoldipine was rather high, what is the advantage of taking nisoldipine?

DEEG:

It is a lower substance load for the patient and maybe when you look on the treatment periods throughout these three treatments you see a decrease in the frequency of side effects. In the first treatment you see the most side effects and in the third treatment period you see much less side effect, so maybe throughout these three treatment periods the patients adapted a little. After all, the question is not finally answered.

Nisoldipine in PTCA patients

B. Höfling[1], A. von Pölnitz[1], R. Meißner[1], M. Stiegelmeier[1], C. Burkhard-Meier[1], Th. von Arnim[2]

[1] Medical Clinic I, University of Munich, Klinikum Großhadern, Munich, FRG and [2] Medical Clinic I, Krankenanstalt Rotes Kreuz, Munich, FRG

Introduction

Vasodilation with drugs such as calcium channel blockers and nitrates (orally, intravenously, or intracoronary) are generally accepted as standard therapy during PTCA [1]). Although their beneficial effects have not clearly been documented by standardized trials, the concept seems convincing since coronary spasm and occlusion are major potential complications of the procedure [2].

Nisoldipine is a new calcium channel blocker from the dihydropyridine group which, in comparison to nifedipine at respective doses, has a high vasodilating capacity without negative inotropic effects [3]. Consequently, it could be useful as adjunctive therapy during PTCA.

Methods

We investigated the action of intravenous (i.v.) Nisoldipine (2 µg/kg given vor 5 min followed by 0.2 µg/kg for 15 min (directly before the beginning of the PTCA procedure) on the hemodynamics of the systemic, pulmonary, and coronary circulation (Fig. 1) in 30 patients, 20 of whom were orally pretreated with Nifedipine, 10 mg every 8 h for at least 24 h. All patients had single vessel disease with the following vessel distribution: Left anterior descending (n = 19), circumflex (n = 4), and right coronary artery (n = 7). The coronary circulation was measured in five patients.

Statistical analysis was performed using the SPSS program with unifactoral variance analysis, Studtent's t-test, and the Kolmogorov-Smirnov test to study drug effect as well as differences between the groups with and without oral calcium channel blocker pre-treatment.

Results

There was a slight but statistically significant increase in heart rate seen in the group without, as well as in the group with oral nifedipine pretreatment (Fig. 1a). In addition, both groups showed a slight, but again significant decrease in systolic blood pressure (Fig. 1b) and increase in cardiac index (Fig. 1c) and, consequently, a decrease in systemic restistance (Fig. 1d). Despite oral Nifedipine pretreatment, left

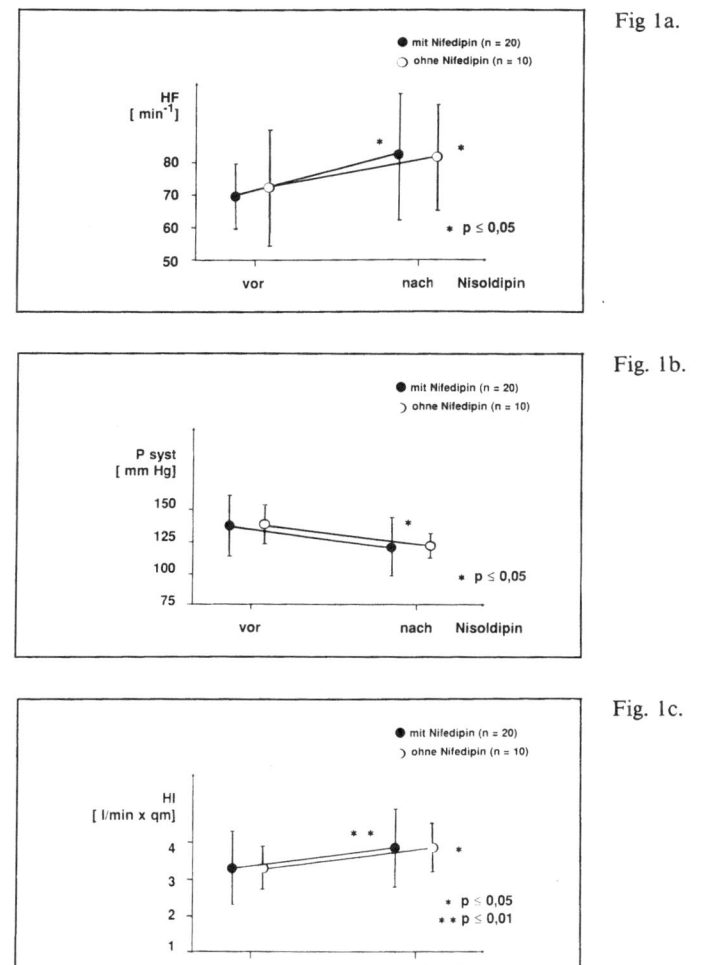

Fig 1a.

Fig. 1b.

Fig. 1c.

Fig. 1d.

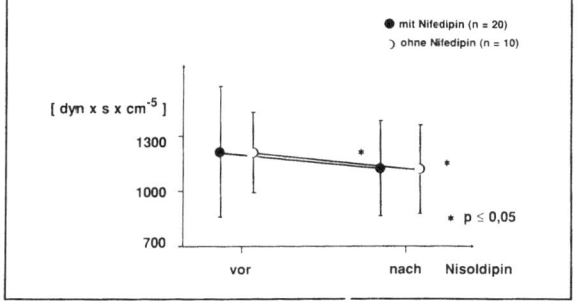

Fig. 1a—d. Comparison of the effects of Nisoldipine infusion (see text for dosage) on heart rate (1a), systolic blood pressure (1b), cardiac index (1c), an systemic vascular resistance (1d) in 20 patients with, and 10 patients without, oral Nifedipine pre-treatment.

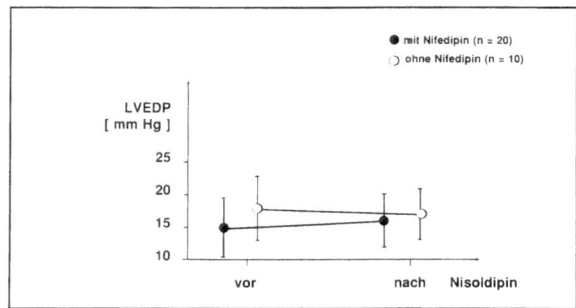

Fig 2a.

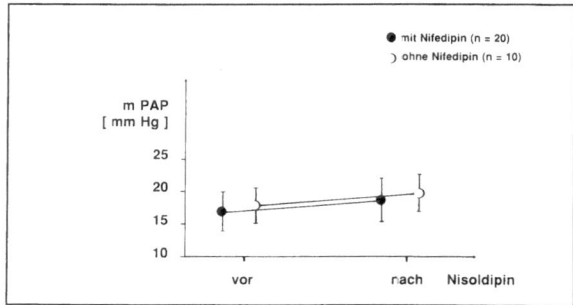

Fig. 2b.

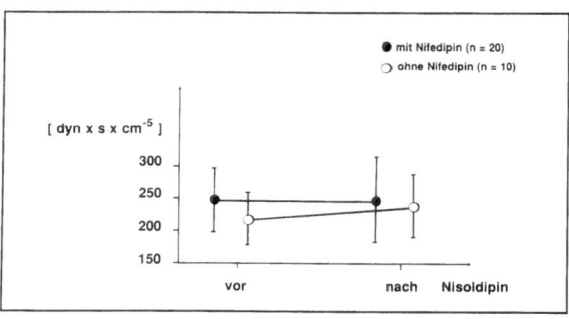

Fig. 2c.

Fig. 2. Comparison of the effects of Nisoldipine infusion on left ventricular end diastolic pressure (2a), pulmonary pressure (2b), and pulmonary vascular resistance (2c) in 20 patients with, and 10 patients without oral Nifedipine pre-treatment.

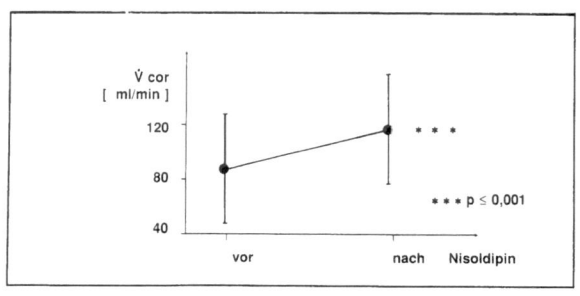

Fig. 3 Effect of Nisoldipine infusion on coronary blood flow in five patients with oral Nifedipine pretreatment.

182

ventricular end-diastolic pressure was not increased by Nisoldipine infusion (Fig. 2a). Pulmonary pressure (Fig. 2b) and resistance (Fig. 2c) were not affected by the dose of i.v. Nisoldpipine used in this study.

The coronary blood flow clearly increased (Fig. 3) due to a considerable decrease in coronary resistance following the Nisoldipine infusion.

Conclusion

This investigation demonstrated that at the selected infusion dosage Nisoldipine has a clear coronary dilating effect without major effect on systemic and pulmonary hemodynamics or on myocardial function. This finding was independent of oral Nifedipine pretreatment, indicating that Nisoldipine dependent coronary vasodilation ist found despite oral nifedipine pretreatment.

References

1. Bussmann WD, Kaltenbach M (1987) Ballondilatation von Herzkranzgefäßen und Herzklappen: Ergebnisse und neuere Entwicklungen. Intensivmed 24: 115—119
2. Cowley MJ, Dorros G, Kelsey SF, Van Raden M, Detre KM (1984) Acute coronary events associated with percutaneous transluminal coronary angioplasty. AJC 53: 12c—16c
3. Daniel WG, Engel HJ, Lichtlen PR (1984) Effects of calcium antagonists on regional myocardial blood flow: Calcium-Antagonismus International. Symposium on Calcium-antagonists; Althaus U, Burckhardt D, Vogt E (eds), Universimed Frankfurt/Main p. 152—161

Author's address:
Prof. Dr. med. B. Höfling
Med. Klinik I
Klinikum Großhadern
Marchioninistr. 15
8000 München 70, FRG

Discussion

LEMMER:

Perhaps you can give your ideas in interpreting that pretreatment with Nifedipine did not influence. Were you at the lower level of the dose response curve with Nifedipine or what is your interpretation of the data?

HÖFLING:

You gave the answer already. The interpretation is that we are very low in the dose response curve, if we use the usual dose of Nifedipine, and we overcome this effect by using Nisoldipine in a dose which is very well tolerated by the systemic circulation. So theoretically, if I could draw a conclusion a little further, I think this could be a good substitute for the usual Nifedipine treatment during PTCA.

KRUCOFF:

Dr. Höfling, do you think there is any possibility this could be a synergistic effect? These are two very different molecules — could they act through different pathways?

HÖFLING:

No, I do not think so, because we have two groups where we have the Nifedipine pretreated plus Nisoldipine and the Nisoldipine group, and from the design of the study I think your question can clearly be excluded.

GOHLKE:

You gave Nisoldipine intravenously?

HÖFLING:

We gave it intravenously while in the process of preparing the PTCA and having these patients in a stable instrumented position.

KARSCH:

Do you think that it would be easier and safer for the patient just to give an intracoronary shot?

HÖFLING:

To speculate, yes. But to be on the cautious side of a clinician working step-by-step, I would say that is the next step, to compare those, and also what we did not do — we did not have a look at how long our effect lasts, does it last one hour, or half an hour, or three hours, we could not look at that because we went on and made a PTCA and many things came together and so we could not check the length of the effect is. But the next step would be to study the long effect of an intravenous dose and then give an intercoronary.

KARSCH:

Yes, the major rationale for using the drug is to prevent spasm and therease coronary blood flow.

DEEG:

The affinity of Nisoldipine to the coronary arteries is in the minimum 10-times higher than that of Nifedipine. When you inject this Nisoldipine into the veins, when you give it intravenously, did you observe some sort of steal phenomenon?

HÖFLING:

No, because we have no possibility to test that. The only indicator for having a steal phenomenon would be the pain of the patient, and if we accept pain as an indicator for steal, we did not see anginal pain in any of the 30 patients.

184

Concluding remarks

This book contains papers and discussions, which are informative and stimulating. They contribute to a better definition of the predisposing conditions for acute ischemic syndromes, thus setting the stage for future research. We have been made more aware that the pathogenesis of acute chronic syndromes is varied and complex.

Intriguing pieces of information are progressively accumulating, which, I am afraid, we are still unable to compose into a coherent picture. I believe that any pathogenetic theory must fit within the following framework:

1) Acute ischemic events are rare in the life of a patient. Rare events cannot be explained by common alterations;
2) Acute coronary occlusion does not necessarily occur only at the site of severe stenosis;
3) Acute coronary syndromes often proceed towards persistent coronary occlusion in an intermittent pattern — a sort of "staccato" phenomenon.

The identification of these problems will inspire "ad hoc" research, and major breakthroughs in our understanding are likely to occur over the next few years.

A. Maseri, London